# Gut Feelings
## the inside story

**Olga Sheean**

Published by InsideOut Media

Published in Canada by InsideOut Media
info@insideoutmedia.net

Cover design, illustrations and layout by Lewis Evans
lewis@lewisevans.net

ISBN 978-1-928103-01-1

# Gut Feelings
## the inside story

# Contents

# Introduction

Like many good stories, this one came about as a result of a 'guy-meets-girl' scenario—but with an unusual twist. I once had a boyfriend who worked odd hours and tended to neglect his health, often eating a big dinner late at night and then going straight to bed. It occurred to me that his body probably wasn't too happy about this and that it must be frustrating for it not to be heard, despite the many symptoms it created to try to get his attention. So I wrote him a letter from his liver—and, boy, did that liver have a lot to say. Years of stored-up anger, resentment and frustration poured out, with scalding invectives and none-too-subtle suggestions as to how things could be improved in that department.

The liver finally got its say and it felt good; it managed to negotiate some cut-backs and there was a truce for a while. Problem was, all the other organs wanted their say then, too, so I couldn't stop there. The pancreas had no sweet things to say about my boyfriend's cravings for sugar; the heart monopolized a good four pages with its appeal for forgiveness and a deep need for meaningful connection; and the intestines went on at length about how much crap they'd had to handle over the years. All in all, it was a massive and hugely enlightening venting process that made me realize just how much our bodies have to say.

Once the various organs and body systems had come to life, of course, they had no intention of retreating back into obscurity. They asserted themselves and took root in my world, evolving into quirky, colourful characters with their own dysfunction, neediness, crises, in-fighting and all the other good things that humans do so well.

Almost all the processes described in this book are based on fact, although not all of them follow the conventional way of thinking, regarding certain bodily functions. For some of the lesser-known physiological truths, I am grateful to the late Frank Ludde—a masterful metabolic therapist who understood the body like no one else I've ever met. If he were alive today, Frank would be happy to know that the body had finally found a stronger voice—and that it had fun doing it. The body likes nothing better than a good belly laugh to lighten things up and freshen our perspective.

The combination of humour, drama, fact and insights in this book is designed to enlighten and entertain, while hopefully also inspiring you to listen to what your body has to say—and to let it take you on a rather special journey of self-discovery. The body is really the only reliable roadmap we get in life; learning how to read it and to interpret the various signs along the way is the most powerful way to get in touch with who you really are. Have a word with your heart about that one and it will soon set you straight.

But be warned: once you open that door, there'll be a chorus of voices urgently clamouring to be heard. Are you ready to hear what your body has to say?

—Olga Sheean, Italy, November 2008

# 1
# Girls go gastric

The hot tarmac makes a faint hissing sound as the two women glide along the path by the water, tanned calves glistening in the sunshine and ponytails swinging to the beat. The rhythmic hum of their Rollerblades blends into the lunchtime buzz: kids playing on the grass, dogs barking, and joggers on cellphones breathlessly coordinating their agendas. Sally and Cynthia are focused, downloading data and cleansing their minds as they weave their way through the tapestry of bodies strolling along the shore. They're like a complementary yin-yang symbol—one lean and pale-skinned, the other solid and African-dark.

"How's work, Cynth?" says Sally, cheeks glowing from the gentle sea breeze. "I haven't seen you since you got promoted to... what was it again? Chief side-kick to the Director of Artistic Worship?"

"More like chief hand-holder," says Cynthia, laughing her deep, throaty laugh. "We've had six exhibitions in a row and I haven't had a breather since Christmas. He can't seem to make a single decision on his own. How he ever got to the top is a mystery to me."

"Sounds as if you could be doing his job for him."

"I *am* doing his job for him. I'm just not getting paid for the privilege. What about you, Sal. What's new with you and Jake?"

"Oh, nothing much."

"Uh oh. I don't like the sound of that. What's up, girl? Spill."

"I think I've been wasting my time, Cynthia. It started out so well. We had so much fun at the beginning. He was funny and generous... but now, I dunno."

"What do you mean, you don't know?" Cynthia slows and looks over at Sally. "You love this guy. What's going on?"

"Oh, he just seems to have turned into a complacent blob.

He has no idea what it means to be fit and healthy, and he shows no sign of becoming enlightened any time soon."

"Not everyone's as health-conscious as you, Sal. Are you sure you're not being too hard on him? Or maybe giving him the six-month Sally shuffle?" She points at a vacant park bench. "Here. Sit."

They flop onto the bench, legs extended, Rollerblades standing to attention. Cynthia takes a water bottle from her backpack and drinks lustily.

Sally looks at her, bemused. "What are you talking about?"

"You always do this. Soon as the guy starts getting too close, you find all kinds of things wrong with him and call it off. He's too fat, too serious, too sex-starved, too caught up in his work, too gorgeous for his own good..."

Sally frowns. "Well, he is! Not too gorgeous but too overweight, anyway, and he's no fun any more. He just seems so... settled, as if he doesn't have to work at the relationship any more. I've been conquered and now he can sit back and just enjoy all the perks of coupledom."

"Sounds good to me. Did it occur to you that maybe he's happy with the way things are, happy with himself?"

"Well, if he is, he shouldn't be. He needs work."

"Sal, he's not a run-down old building that you can upgrade and re-model, you know. And you can't treat him like a client, either, and turn him into a raw foodie who jogs 20 miles a day. This is a man you said you loved. If you don't love him, why are you still with him?"

"I keep hoping he'll change, I suppose." Cynthia rolls her eyes. "I know, I know. But isn't it healthy to grow in relationships? I mean, surely that's what they're for. He just seems to have ground to a halt. He's got his job, his woman and he's just coasting and indulging in life without growing in any way—except above the belt. Ugh."

"Whereas you *have* been growing, of course. Growing in leaps and bounds and leaving him miles behind, right?

"At least I've kept in shape and haven't let myself go all flabby.

How can men get away with being any old shape when their woman must be svelte and shapely? Is there such a worldwide shortage of decent, intelligent, self-respecting males that women have to settle for such inferior goods?"

"Dunno, but I think it's interesting that you keep attracting the same kind of men."

"What do you mean?"

"Well, none of them are what you want and something always goes screwy after about three months. Maybe it's something to do with you, girl. After all, you're the common denominator here. Why do you think you keep attracting these men?"

"Why did I ever bother going to a shrink when I had you for a friend?" She pulls her water bottle from her backpack and takes a long drink.

"My thoughts exactly. So...? Stop avoiding the question."

"Okay, okay. I have been trying to figure that out but I don't know why I attract them, if I do..." She stares at the passersby, watching a mother hauling a screaming two-year-old by the arm as he struggles to get free.

"Maybe start using your heart instead of your head. Scary foreign territory, I know." She looks meaningfully at Sally, waiting for her to refocus. "Look, we all play different roles, right? You're the care-taking kind—showing people how to get healthy, eat better, all that stuff. So it makes sense that you'd attract men who want someone to take care of them and don't take responsibility for themselves. But men hate it when you try to change them and it never works. So you both end up feeling like victims and nobody gets what they want."

"Okay, so what's the answer?"

"You, of course. Maybe if you start changing the way you relate to him, things will change."

"Like what, though? You mean stop taking care of him?"

"That and looking at what you need to change in yourself and how you may not be fully committed to you."

"But you know I—"

"Yeah, but that's all body stuff. What about going deeper?

What about all the emotional stuff, the deeper intimacy you're always talking about? You can't have that unless you're willing to go there yourself."

"But—"

"Look..." She sits sideways on the bench to face Sally. "Just think of the things you find hard to do in relationships and you'll find your answer there."

Sally is about to respond when her cellphone buzzes in her knapsack. "That will be Jake. He said he'd call to arrange dinner." She looks questioningly at Cynthia, who gestures at her to take the call.

Sally rummages in the front pocket of her rucksack and pulls out the pulsating phone. "Hello? Oh, hi Jake... Yes, fine, yes. What time? Oh, I see ...6.30, then. My place. Yeah, okay. Thanks. Bye."

She hands up, shoves the phone back into her rucksack and grimaces. "This is hopeless. He's going for a drink with Charlie before we go out for dinner. He'll have a couple of beers at the pub then he'll have wine with dinner... God, I find that such a turn-off!"

Cynthia looks at her watch. "Listen, I've gotta get moving but there's one other thing I can suggest..." She starts rummaging in her back pack. "Maybe, if you're clever, you can get him to start thinking differently—while you work on yourself, of course—and have a little fun while you're at it."

"Oh, no. No more of your crazy ideas. I remember the last time you suggested something creative. I've never been so mortified in my life."

"Yes you have. You've been mortified lots. That's part of the problem, you know—caring too much what other people think of you. It stops you from being outrageous, having a bit of fun. Anyway, this is much more subtle." She continues rummaging in her back pack, unzipping side pockets and pulling out lipstick, tampons, perfume, pens, wallet, cell phone, mustard spray, address book... until finally.... "Ah, here it is." She holds up a small clear sachet of dark-brown powder. "Something special from my herbal witchdoctor friend Dean, guaranteed to have an immediate and powerful effect."

"What?" Sally looks at her, horrified. "The Dean who ended up in hospital with that funny skin disease?" She makes a face. "I don't think so, Cynthia..."

"It's perfectly harmless." She waves the sachet back and forth and drops it into Sally's lap. "Would I give you something iffy?"

"Yes."

"Look, knowing you, you'll have a hard time getting out of this relationship even if it's not what you want. You're such a sucker for punishment. This is a make-or-break moment. You need to take drastic measures—mostly with yourself, but this could help shift things. I call it my herbal dynamite. Just mix it into his coffee and he'll never know. Really gets things moving. Speaking of which..." She starts stuffing everything back into her backpack.

"I don't think this is a good idea, Cynthia," says Sally, seriously. She picks up the sachet and holds it up to the light. "It's a laxative, right? Fast-acting, I suppose?"

"Oh, yeah. Turbo-charged." Cynthia closes the last zipper, gets up and hoists her knapsack onto her back. "Come on, Sal, let's go." She sets off along the path, motioning at Sally to follow. "Pop that thing in your pack. You've got plenty of time to think about it before dinner. And stop worrying!"

# 2
# Men at work

Jake is musing about life and doesn't hear the first knock. Swivelling lazily from side to side in his plush leather chair, he props his feet up on the windowsill and sighs deeply. The afternoon sun is streaming in through the floor-to-ceiling windows of his office and all is tidy on his polished desk with matching pen-holder, fancy phone and IN-tray. He's studying his reflection in the glass and sees a 35-year-old top marketing executive, with dark unruly hair, tanned skin, crisp white shirt, funky tie and expensive black suit. Not bad. Not bad at all... He's just about to reach for his coffee mug, when there's another knock at his door.

"Yes! You may enter the kingdom of Heaven—IF you bear tidings of joy... or at least a few good jokes."

The door opens and a perky young woman sweeps into the office, carrying a large red folder. She is confident, slim, with wavy auburn hair, a touch of make-up and dressed in a well-cut dark-green suit over a cream V-neck clingy top. She places the folder on Jake's desk and laughs.

"Well, I'm not sure how amusing you'll find these, Your Holiness, but I've prepared the campaign proposal for Cressing & Blake. Contract's in there too." She turns to go.

"Thanks, Jen. I'm sure it's all in order... always is..." He pauses, looking at her quizzically.

"What's up, Jake. You don't look your usual ebullient self. Trouble with the boss?"

"Ah, depends which boss you mean—the big cheese upstairs or the woman who's trying to run my life." He pauses. "You remember Sally—the woman I met at the office party?"

"Slim, short blond hair, green eyes, good legs, wearing The Black Dress?" Jake nods, smiling.

"No, don't remember her at all." Jennifer laughs heartily. "Okay, okay. Say no more. Woman trouble. I get the picture." She grins mischievously, rubs her hands together gleefully and plops into a chair in front of Jake's desk. "Time for a man-to-woman talk, I think, don't you?"

"Yes!" He pauses, uncertain, with a look of mock-angst. "You mean her and me or you and me?"

"Both," says Jennifer, all businesslike. "But we need to do a practice run. First things first. Do you love her?"

"Yes, I do. I do love her. Phew." He smiles, surprised at his own reaction. "I didn't realize I knew. That's a relief ...I think."

"Okay, okay, good. More importantly, though, do you *like* her?"

"Ah. Sneaky. I wasn't ready for that one. Um, not sure, really. I like many things about her but I don't think I like the way she's treating me or behaving towards me..."

"Ummm... that sounds like a no—provisionally, anyway. Right. Good to get that cleared up. Now, what do you do around here when something happens that you don't like—like when that silly cow from accounting short-changed you by $2,000 on your end-of-year bonus?

"Well, I tell her to take a hike up to the Yukon, with all her deformed, mentally retarded relatives, and that if she ever even thinks of siphoning bucks from my bonus again I'll ram two bottles of white-out up her prim little nostrils and decorate her earlobes with the heavy-duty staple gun."

"Which is macho-speak for what, exactly?"

"Oh, something like, 'dear Ms Partridge, sorry to disturb you but you seem to have mislaid a few dollars of mine and I've just come to collect them, if you don't mind. Thank you so much'."

"Okay, so you'd let her know it didn't work for you, this egregious, totally unacceptable behaviour of hers. And you wouldn't let her get away with it again, right?" Jennifer sits back, arms folded, looking smug.

"Yeah, right." He pauses, looking at her uncertainly. "That's it? That's your priceless womanly advice?"

"What else is there?" Jennifer looks at him in mock innocence. "You've got to tell this woman that it's not okay to push you around ...unless you enjoy being pushed around and then moaning about it." She raises her eyebrows questioningly, gets up and crisply brushes her short skirt, as if to dispel any lingering male vibes.

"I suppose you're right." Jake looks lost. "But what if she doesn't like what I say or the way I say it?"

"Tough. Let her walk, then. State your terms. If she doesn't like 'em, better to get out now than to tough it out for 35 years and end up a hen-pecked, beaten old fart in fluffy slippers and flannel dressing-gown, being force-fed all kinds of nasty healthfoods, never allowed alcohol and told what to wear every day."

Jake looks horrified. "Jen, please, do you have to be so graphic? How do you know all that stuff anyway? You barely spoke to her at the party."

"I know the type."

"The type?"

"She's the cucumber-and-salmon-on-dry-crispbread type," says Jennifer, authoritatively. "One glass of chilled white wine, absolutely no deep-fried finger food, and half a centimetre of extra-dark organic chocolate at exactly 4pm every day." She looks at him challengingly.

"And I thought all you girls stuck together."

"No point in prolonging the agony—for you or for her. You've got to love, like *and* respect each other, otherwise it'll never work. Be honest with her, Jake. It's the only way." She turns on her three-inch heel, blows him a cheeky kiss and waltzes out the door, shutting it softly behind her.

Jake sits absolutely still for a full minute. "Shit." He reaches for the phone and speed-dials. "Charlie? Listen, any chance you could knock off early? I'm heading down to the pub now... Yeah? Great. See you there in ten."

★ ★ ★

Just after 4.30pm, Charlie was one of only three customers occupying the tables along the walls. "Hey, buddy, you made it. Wasn't sure you could get away early." Jake slapped Charlie on

15

the shoulder and sat down opposite him.

"Yeah. Been a slow day. The whole damn month has been slow."

"Trouble at the plant?" Jake waved at the waitress behind the counter and pointed to Charlie's beer.

"More cutbacks. Output is down. You know the story."

"But they'll always need a production manager, right?"

"Yeah …unless they merge with the sister company up north." Charlie shrugged. "I'm casting around, just in case."

"Right." Jake smiled at the waitress, nodding his thanks as she placed a beer on a mat in front of him. "Maybe a move would be good."

"Yeah." Charlie took a swig of beer.

"How's Deirdre? Haven't seen her for ages."

"Great. She's great. How are things with you and Sally?"

"We're having fun. It's good. Hey, did you see the game last night? Wasn't that a lousy break for McKinney?"

"Are you kidding? He was asking for it. You could see it coming."

Jake knocked back half his beer and licked the froth from his lips. He checked his watch and glanced at the TV mounted over the bar. "We can catch the highlights at 5. You in a rush to get home?"

"Nah. I've got time." They drained their glasses and moved to the bar stools facing the TV. "Another beer?"

"Sure, why not."

# 3
# In digestion

The vast, dimly lit chamber was a hive of frenzied activity. At its centre stood Sam Stomach, looking apoplectic. His face almost as red as the curved chamber's walls, Sam was glaring at the main entry valve. "What the heck is that muck coming down now?" he demanded of no one in particular. "Surely he can't be having another one of those greasy heart-burners that keep us up all night, can he? I've barely cleared the decks after that little mid-afternoon snack of chocolate and coffee, and now he's guzzling again. We need Burnie and his team down here, fast! Sylvie, call Des and get him to send Burnie over."

"I'm on it," said Sylvie, plucking a round, pulsating cell phone from the wall. "Don't get so worked up, dear, please. We'll sort it out." The phone pulsed twice, glowing brightly, before it was picked up.

"Des Dispatch. What can I do for you?"

"Des, it's Sylvie Stomach. Sam needs Burnie and his team over here right now."

"Okay, Sylvie. What exactly is the situation?"

"Well, it's looking rather explosive, with gas building up already. We just got word in from Command Central that there's a storm brewing and we're looking at high winds—from here right down through Colon County, Rectum Region and out by Anus Alley. It doesn't look good."

"Right-oh. Burnie's on his way," said Des, hanging up.

"Why is that guy always late when we need him?" said Sam, pacing back and forth, exasperated. "Doesn't he know that as soon as we get food in here he has to be ready with the hydrochloric acid? How many times... Burnie! What the hell took you so long to get here?"

"Keep yer hair on, Sam." Burnie, a short, stocky man with

red hair and freckles, appeared behind him, dressed in a bright-yellow jumpsuit and protective helmet with a transparent visor. He's carrying a large canister of hydrochloric acid over his shoulder and is followed by a team carrying hoses, shovels and other tools. "Me and the crew only got off the late-afternoon shift a few hours ago and we weren't expecting anything else to go down for a while. We need our shut-eye, too, ye know."

"Well don't waste precious time with excuses," said Sam. "Get your men to work straight away. If any more of this protein goes down undigested, we're toast. We'll be up all night with gale-force winds blowing right into the middle of tomorrow. I don't know what's going on up there. Too much talk and smooching, if you ask me. The stuff didn't even come down properly chewed, so not even the starches have been broken down. It's a mess. It all has to be converted into liquid or else—"

"Yeah, yeah, I know," said Burnie. "Guys, over here with that hose. You know the drill. Soak down this stuff here for a few minutes and then get yer shovels. We'll need to mix it in manually to make sure it's all broken down. George, watch the levels, there."

"Yeah, boss." George Gastric, in charge of gastric juices, starts pouring measured doses of a thin, colourless liquid onto the mass of food.

"What's that, George?" says Ivan, an intern on Burnie's team.

"This here's a mixture of pepsin, which breaks proteins down into smaller, more manageable bits; rennet, which helps digest milk proteins; and mucin, which protects the walls from that hydrochloric acid that Burnie's using to—" He's interrupted by his boss.

"George, how much time we got till the other guys move in?"

"About thirty minutes, I reckon."

"What other guys?" said Sylvie. "You don't think...?"

"Well, if we don't get this cleared up fast enough, we're looking at a possible invasion of the Bacteria Brigade, which is not good. If they get their mitts on all this putrefying material they'll have a field day. And if that happens, well, you know what His Lordship did last time..."

"Oh, no. Not the Pepto Bismol?" said Sylvie, chewing her lip.

"Yeah," said Burnie. "An antacid's the last thing we want. We might need some help from Pete."

"I'll call him," said Sylvie, reaching for the cell phone again.

"This is Pete Pancreas. What's up?"

"Oh, blood pressure, pulse rate and a few other things... Pete, it's Sylvie. We need some more ammo here. Burnie says we're going to need more help further down in the duodenum. Can you arrange for some heavy-duty enzyme action?"

"Which enzymes do you need?" said Pete. "Are they for simple or complex starches, and are we looking at heavy proteins and fats too?"

"Well, I'm not sure, exactly..." said Sylvie. She cupped her hand over the receiver and yelled to Sam, "Did anyone get a look at the menu?"

"No," said Burnie. "We'll do that right now, but tell Pete to send in all he's got anyway. We're going to need Polly Peptides—"

"Who's she, boss?" asked Ivan.

Irritated, Burnie paused to explain. "Polly breaks down the protein into lots of smaller particles—peptides. It's a bit like making kindling from firewood: ye can't light a fire using just the large raw logs. Then the food goes into the first part of Highway 22—"

"What's Highway 22?" says Ivan.

"It's a 22-foot-long highway that runs the length of Colon County, and the first part is called the duodenum, where most of the digestion takes place." Ivan is scribbling furiously as Burnie keeps an eye on George and the rest of the team. "Carbohydrates are broken down into simpler sugars, proteins to amino acids, and fats to fatty acids and glycerol. Then Lily Liver's department sends in Brendan Bile via his own personal duct, and Pete Pancreas sends the other enzymes directly into the intestines—as he's about to do now."

"But what about—"

"Not now, Ivan. I'm far too busy. You'll just have to watch and take notes."

Burnie turned back to Sylvie. "Get Pete to send in everything."

"Right," said Sylvie, turning back to the phone. "Pete, send us the works. We'll find out about the menu right away. Thanks."

"No problem, Sylvie. Hey, you know me: breakdown is what I do best, especially under pressure."

"Oh, please, Pete, how many more times are you going to use that one?" Sylvie shakes her head, smiling as she hangs up, and turns to watch Burnie and his crew. They're all working feverishly with their shovels, turning over the food and hosing it down with hydrochloric acid. Bits of cookies and toast, melted chocolate, fragments of fries, chunks of meat and blobs of ketchup could be seen in the mess. Burnie is standing off to one side, chewing on a matchstick and giving orders. Sylvie could see him grimace behind his visor as the fermenting mass bubbled and belched noxious gases into the air. The mound of food was slowly beginning to break down and was accumulating in a pool at Burnie's feet. He looked down and frowned. There were still large chunks of undigested material floating around in the liquid and the level was rising rapidly.

"George!" he yelled. "This isn't working. Get on to CC about that menu right now. We need to know what else is coming down if we're to stand a chance of getting on top of it all."

"Right, boss," said George, squelching knee-deep through the debris and heading for the cell phone on the wall. He pushed the red button and got straight through to Crystal.

"Command Central. Crystal, here. What can I do for you?"

"It's George Gastric, on the digestive squad—"

"I know who it is, George. You forget that I have neurotransmitters *and* call-display. Now what's the problem? I've been getting signals up here that there's some overload in the works."

"Yes, there is," said George. "We've got a crisis down here and it's not getting any better. We need to know what His Lordship had for dinner, and what else he's planning on having. A forecast would help, though at this stage it's really just a matter of damage control."

"I'll patch you through to E&E, George," said Crystal. "Hang on." There was a click on the line and silence for a moment. Leaning against the wall, George felt a shudder go through the system and groaned. *More food coming down*, he thought. *Just what we need.* He was exhausted and it looked like another long night...

"George, Eyes 'n Ears here. How can we help you?"

"Things aren't looking too good..." said George.

"Well, we know that, George. What do you think we do all day? We can see what's been going down. Now, I gather you want to know the complete menu. Hang on a sec while I just check the memory banks. Okay... Well, for starters, he had an egg mayonnaise, with some little toastie things on the side, and lashings of butter. Then... let me see. He was toying with the idea of the prime rib, but his lady friend managed to dissuade him from that, thank goodness. He finally opted for the burger with fries, more mayo, mustard and ketchup. Not much better, as it turns out."

George groaned again, and wiped his sweating brow with the back of his hand.

"Anything else?" said George, thoroughly depressed.

"Well, let's see..."

"No vegetables, salad or anything like that?" prompted George, already knowing the answer.

"Nope. He's just finishing up the main course, and word is he's planning on having dessert. I'd say you've got about another fifteen minutes before that particular delight hits the system. Doesn't sound like his lady friend has much say in this one. She tried, though, poor girl. Anyway, we'll call you as soon as we have the details but, knowing His Lordship, I'd say it's a fairly safe bet that it's going to be rich, creamy and loaded with sugar. Oh, I almost forgot. He's already had three glasses of vino, on top of the beer he had earlier. Rather you than me, pal. Good luck."

George hung up the phone and let out a weary sigh. He felt old. *I've been doing this non-stop for 35 years,* he thought, *and there's no end in sight.* If only he could take a vacation, get some rest with the family and kids, he would soon bounce back to his old, energetic self. Maybe they could go to—

"George! Get over here!" He turned to see Burnie beckoning him over. "We need you. Pete just sent in some action and they're getting to work now. I want you to supervise the lot of them and make sure they cover all the bases. Let them know what exactly went down. I'll be over here working on the valve system to make sure everything's ready for dispatch to Highway 22."

"Okay, guys," said George, turning to the crew. "Here's the scoop. We're looking at heavy animal proteins, simple starches, animal fats, alcohol, food colourings and some preservatives. No need to worry about the last three—that's not our problem— but we need to get to work on the proteins, starches and fats, pronto—and prepare for sugar and dairy to follow. God knows that's the worst combination, but His Lordship, in his infinite wisdom... Anyway, I need you, Peggy Protease, Anton Amylase, Lyle Lipase—and, yeah, you too, Celine Cellulase—all working double shifts, with back-up. And where's Larry Lactase? I need him to be ready to break down the dairy."

"He's off sick, George," said one of the crew. "Too much overtime lately."

George shook his head in weary resignation. "You'd think that, with all the congestion that it causes, His Lordship would avoid dairy," he muttered to himself. "But, no, it tastes good and that's all that matters. Out of sight, out of mind. Typical. Well, he'll be paying for it tomorrow morning..." He sighed and turned back to the enzyme squad who were busy loading their spray guns.

"You guys should have been here before all this started," George said, irritably. "We shouldn't have to call you in."

"Hey, don't you start on us," said Peggy, pulling off her protective goggles. "We're just about worn out with all this over-activity. How much do you think the Pancreas Patrol can take, anyway? We were told that we wouldn't have to work more than three or four shifts a day, max. But in the last three-to-four months, we've been working practically around the clock. So don't give us a hard time. Much more of this, and we'll all be thinking of packing it in. No more action. *Finito. Nada* ...unless His Lordship turns over a new leaf and gives us all a break."

"Okay, Peggy, sorry," said George. "We're all overworked here and none of us gets compensated for overtime, so I know how you feel. Let's just do the best we can, and when this crisis is under control, maybe we can have a union meeting to try and work out a new schedule. Okay?"

"Well, all right, then," said Peggy, mumbling to herself as she put her goggles back on. "But someone had better make sure that our needs get met because after this shift we want a *holiday*."

A sound like rolling thunder suddenly came from above. Everyone stops working and looks up only just in time to see a massive boulder come hurtling down the chute towards them at top speed. Dropping shovels and hoses, they fling themselves off to the side. But Ivan and two other interns are not quite quick enough. Ivan is pinned to the ground, his arm under the boulder, and the other two are sent flying from a glancing impact. Within seconds, George and the rest of his team have rolled the boulder off Ivan and pulled him clear. Ivan's arm is broken, but his co-workers appear unhurt, though dazed.

"What… what was that?" Ivan stood up on shaky legs, cradling his broken arm. Peggy tore a strip off her loose cheesecloth shirt and began making him a makeshift sling.

"That, Ivan, was a fine example of 'out of sight, out of mind'— pure indulgence with no consideration for the consequences."

"But what exactly *was* it?"

"It was a lump of unchewed meat," said George, shaking his head angrily. "How can he swallow such massive chunks of food without even chewing them? Doesn't he know that we can't cope with this kind of thing? This is going to set us back by at least another two hours."

He sent Ivan off to the infirmary with his two co-workers and told them to get checked for concussion. With a heavy sigh, he turned back to the crew.

"We're going to need the heavy-duty drilling equipment to break up this lot. It's going to cause some fairly serious gurgling, gas and acid regurgitation, but that can't be helped. It's the very least he deserves…"

The cell phone rang and George went over to answer it.

"George, it's E&E here again. The good news is that his Lordship is having apple pie with ice cream, followed by coffee."

"That's the good news?" said George.

"Yeah. The bad news is that his lady friend has just slipped something into his coffee, and it's not an aphrodisiac."

"What the heck is it, then?" said George, running his fingers through his hair.

"Well, if I were you down there, I'd clear the decks. Things could accelerate a little, if you know what I mean."

"Oh, no," groaned George. A laxative was all they needed after this huge meal. "How'd she manage that, anyway? Those things taste awful. Didn't the Taste Buddies catch it?"

"Well, they did, which is how I got to hear about it, but His Lordship has no frame of reference for this kind of thing so he didn't know what it was. Plus it's got a bitter taste like coffee, so he probably wouldn't have noticed it."

"Great," said George. "Just great."

"Look at it this way, George. Better out than in, right? Take care."

"Yeah. Thanks a lot."

Hanging up the phone, George Gastric looked around for his boss. Burnie was busy adjusting the valves at the end of the corridor. He looked frustrated. George walked over, not looking forward to breaking the news.

"Burnie, we've got a problem..."

"Yeah, I know that, George. You're supposed to be working on it," said Burnie.

"No, I mean another problem," said George. "A worse one."

Burnie straightened up and looked at George. "Well? Spit it out, man. I haven't got all day."

"Well, the good news is that we won't need to do any more work here tonight. The bad news is that we can expect an attack of the runs in the next few hours. There's some fast-acting laxative coming down so all this work will be wasted."

"Shit!" said Burnie.

"Exactly," said George.

"Okay, sound the Red Alert," said Burnie, "and remind CC to alert Colon County of what to expect."

"But what if—?"

"Just do it, George. Now!"

"Right," said George, turning on his heel and heading for the alarm. He hated this part. Now all hell would break loose and it would be chaos for hours. Not to mention what his Lordship might get up to, if the last time was anything to go by. He reached up for the big red lever, and pulled down firmly. Immediately, a deafening siren echoed throughout the chamber, stopping everyone in their tracks. With his hands over his ears, George gestured for the crews to gather up their tools and head home.

Sam turned towards him, a mixture of disgust and rage contorting his face. "And who gave you the order to do that?" he shouted above the din.

"Burnie, Sam. He had no choice. We're expecting the runs in a few hours. We need to clear the decks."

"That's your excuse for not being able to handle the job?" said Sam, sarcastically, reaching over and reversing the lever.

"Sam, a little more respect and appreciation might be in order here," Burnie said from behind him. "Perhaps you forget that, without us, no food would ever get digested—which means that none of you would get fed, let alone have a job. No nutrients would be absorbed, and vitamin and mineral deficiencies would set in. Very soon, there would be an iron shortage, and we'd have the nails complaining about ridges, the scalp moaning about hair loss, and everyone going around dizzy, pale and tired. We'd have a mutiny on our hands in Immune Inc., and—"

"All right, all right!" said Sam. "Just get the hell out of here and give me some peace."

"No problem, Sam. Just put the alarm back on. You know the rules."

Sam reached up, his face a grimace, and pulled down hard on the lever.

# 4
# Tummy trouble

"Jake, what's wrong?" Sally said, leaning over the table towards him. "You look terrible."

"I've suddenly got an awful headache," said Jake, rubbing his temples. "It feels as if the hunchback of Notre Dame is using my skull as a bell tower."

"Must have been something you ate. Maybe we should get you home so you can rest. Let's just pay the bill and go."

"Well, okay, if you don't mind," said Jake feebly. "My stomach does feel a little queasy. Perhaps I overdid it with the dessert..."

*And the wine, and the French fries, and the coffee*, thought Sally, ruefully, picking up her bag.

"There must be some vast cosmic injustice at work, here," said Jake.

"What do you mean?" Sally looked worried. He couldn't possibly know about the powder, could he? He'd been in the men's washroom when she slipped it in...

"Why on earth am I smitten with a woman whose metabolism works at the speed of light, when mine doesn't even wake up until late evening? You can eat whatever you want and it doesn't affect you."

"There's no big mystery, you know," said Sally. "You eat like a Neanderthal, sit at your desk all day, and then expect to be trim and fit. You might want to think about adopting a 21st century diet and exercising occasionally."

Jake sighed. "Merciless, just merciless, even when I'm dying."

He put some money on the table and she took his arm as they headed for the door.

"A nice hot bath and an early night and you'll be fine in the morning," she said soothingly.

"God," he said. "It feels as if there's a war going on in my insides. Maybe I should take some antacid or something."

"No, Jake, I don't think that would help," said Sally, calmly, as they approached the car. "You might just have to let it run its course. Why don't you give me the keys and I'll drive."

"But what if it's food poisoning?" said Jake, his face pale as he handed her the keys. "I could be very sick. Maybe I should tell the waiter that there was something bad in the food." He turned half-heartedly towards the restaurant, but Sally steered him back towards the car.

"Come on, let's just get you home."

She helped him into the front seat, cursing Cynthia. *You and your magic potions!*

"I'm sure it's just because you ate too much," said Sally, getting in the driver's side. "Maybe you need to burn off a few calories—do something physical."

"Right now, I'll settle for all the mod cons, comforts and pampering I can get," said Jake, rubbing his distended stomach.

"Not feeling too amorous, then, I take it," said Sally, putting on her seat belt and turning on the ignition.

"Just take me home, Sal," said Jake dolefully. "Get me back to my nice, warm bed, close to my nice modern bathroom, and I'll be your slave for life."

"Deal," said Sally.

# 5
# Colon chaos

Frederick Fungus was in his element—literally. "Boy," he said to his fellow-fungi, "that was some decadent stuff His Lordship sent down last night. I've never had such a delectable feast of fermenting sugars, starches and undigested proteins in all my anaerobic life." There were grunts of agreement from his cohorts who were lying, heaped on top of each other along a cul-de-sac off Highway 22, in various stages of stupor. Feeling well sated, Frederick too lay back against his spongy villi-couch and stared lazily up at the ceiling. "These villi need some work," he reflected, half to himself. "They're getting a bit deflated—not as spongy as they used to be. I wonder if Crystal in Command Central knows about it."

"Oh, she knows all about it," said Candice Candida, licking the remains of some tasty sugar morsels off her fingers. "She just can't get the message through to the left side of the brain."

"What's the problem?" said Frederick. "Why can't she get through?"

"You should know the answer to that," said Candice. "After all, you're the reason for it."

"What do you mean?" said Frederick, half sitting up. "I'm just doing what comes naturally—gorging myself on all this excess junk down here. Why is it *my* fault?"

"You and your gang spend all day lounging around on your villi, and nobody can get any work done with you in the way," said Candice. "You've flattened half of them," she said, pointing to the collapsed cone-shaped villi, "and you've damaged the walls with your brawling. These things used to be lovely and clean, upright and springy, but nothing gets absorbed now, thanks to you lot, and the forecast doesn't look good. There's a brain fog moving in, with some occasional bright spells, but the outlook is mainly cloudy for the next few hours. That'll be followed by gusts of noxious wind and a ridge of high pressure up north at Fore Head—"

"Hold on a minute!" said Frederick, trying to get up but too tired to make it. "What about you and your lot. You cause just as much gas and confusion. Not to mention all the congestion in Colon County and the cravings for chocolate chip cookies, cheeseca—"

"What is going on here?"

Frederick and Candice turned to see the tall, formidable figure of Ace Acidophilus, standing with his hands on his hips, glaring at them both.

"Look at this mess! Didn't I tell you lot to clear out of here and not come back?" said Ace, striding over to Frederick and stabbing a finger into his pudgy belly. "I warned you that if I found you loitering here again I would take serious action."

"What action?" said Frederick, finally managing to get to his feet. "You're completely outnumbered this time, in case you hadn't noticed," he said, gesturing to his snoring companions.

"You do nothing but cause havoc with these sickening bingeing parties," said Ace.

"We *like* causing havoc, Ace," said Frederick, belching loudly. "And what, exactly, are you going to do about it? You look pretty defenceless down here all on your owney-oh."

"I've got back-up," said Ace curtly. "There's my team, and Barney Bifidus with his crew, and I can call in Simon Salivarius too, if I need to, not to mention the entire Immune Inc. workforce. We've got entire armies at our disposal, as if you didn't know. So get moving before I get them all over here."

"Oh, very impressive," said Frederick sarcastically. "You're bluffing. They're all off sick or on holiday, otherwise they'd be here with you. So you don't scare me. I'm going back to bed."

"Fine!" said Ace, fuming. "I'll be back." He turned smartly and strode off.

"Oh, make my day!" Frederick yelled after him, before settling back on his villi with his hands behind his head.

"I think we'd better go," said Candice, looking around

nervously. "You know what happened last time. There were billions of them, swarming all over the place. We lost half our crew and—"

"Oh, stop whining, woman," said Frederick. "He doesn't stand a chance against us lot. Last time he was just lucky. His Lordship hadn't been on a binge like this and we were short on numbers. This time, we're ahead of the game and... What's that noise?" He sat up and cocked his head, listening.

"It's them!" said Candice, terrified. "They're back. I'm out of here. You can stay and fight if you want, but I'd prefer to hide out till this is over." She looked around desperately, trying to decide which way to go. If she went north, she might run into trouble from the gastric squad; and if she went south, she could run into heavy traffic at this hour. She froze on the spot, a tingle of dread creeping up her spine. She could see them swarming towards her from both directions. They were surrounded. "He's brought in Immune Inc.," she gasped. "We're done for."

She could hear Ace shouting orders. "Larry, get your crew over here and bring Phil with you." She looked around desperately and made a run for the nearest emergency exit.

"Neutro Phil or Baso Phil?" called back Larry Lymphocyte.

"I don't know," said Ace impatiently. "I don't even know what they do. That's *your* job."

"Well, Neutro Phil's responsible for engulfing bacteria, and Baso Phil's in charge of allergies, bringing in histamine and—"

"Bring both of them, for heaven's sake," shouted Ace, putting on his gloves. "Don't you have a supervisor?"

"'Course we do," said Larry, gesturing to his crew to get ready for action. "But he's busy right now with a problem further north. Anyway, we're in contact," he said, tapping the cell phone strapped to his belt, "and we know what we're doing."

"Good," said Ace, turning back to his own team. "Guys, I want you cleaning up all this debris and taking care of any bacteria lying around. We need to clear the passageway before Sam's shift goes on duty again in the morning."

Suddenly the place was filled with activity. Larry and his

million-strong crew swarmed up the walls and began peeling Frederick's dozing companions off each other. Dazed and still in a stupor from their night's bingeing, they were quickly surrounded. Ace's team was working furiously with long-nozzled vacuum cleaners, scouring debris from the floor and in between the deflated villi.

Within twenty minutes, the frenzy had begun to subside and Ace stood back to survey the situation. Larry joined him, mopping his brow as his team took care of the remaining offenders. "Nice work," said Ace, "but... oh, no, take cover, men! Grab something!"

There was a stampede towards the walls as a huge spasm shook the organism and the ground began to vibrate. In the distance, the sound of thunder could be heard and all heads turned to see what was coming down the pipeline. Grasping for a purchase on the slippery villi, Ace, Larry and their teams hung on for dear life. As the noise grew louder, a strong wind came hurtling down the passageway, threatening to sweep them off their feet.

"Just hold on tight," shouted Ace above the noise. He was sheltering behind a curve in the wall, with his body wedged firmly between two crevices. Bracing himself for the inevitable, he closed his eyes and tried to ignore the stench carried by the strong southwesterly gale.

Suddenly a torrent of putrid brown liquid surged down the passageway, flattening everything in its path and plunging them into darkness. Ace hung on, feeling the suction of the rapidly flowing gunge, and praying that it would not last long. "A hundred thousand curses on His Lordship," he swore. "And his lady friend," he added, remembering the evening news bulletin from Command. "What the hell does he think happens to all that junk he eats? He must think we have a team of fairies down here with magic wands, ready to convert it all into clean, fully combustible, life-enhancing nutrients. Or maybe he just doesn't think at all." He sighed, wondering what to do when the flood was over. It seemed to be lessening, and the wind had dropped. He opened his eyes and peered out from around the villi. The passageway was still half-filled with muck, but the level was quickly dropping and it looked as if it would soon be gone.

He waited, looking around for his crew and Larry. No one was in sight. As the last of the flood drained away, he climbed gingerly down from his hiding place and stepped into the passageway. The air was still putrid, and he held his nose as he cast around for signs of life.

"Larry? Men? Are you dere? Id's Ace," he called out, his nose still firmly plugged. There were muted groans from his left and he turned to see some of his team emerging from between the villi. "Dank goodness," he said, gesturing them over. "Now listen, team," he said, slowly releasing his grip on his nose. "We've got to repopulate this place now that the low-life quota has been reduced. We can't afford to let them get a grip again. Barney, call Crystal and ask her to make sure we get all the support we need from Friendly Flora. And see if there's any sign of things improving, up there."

Barney Bifidus pulled out his cell phone and dialed Command Central. Ace could hear him talking to Crystal as he turned to make sure the area was secured.

"Boss," said Barney, putting away his phone. "Crystal says there's been a new development. It looks like things might be getting better after all."

# 6
# The morning after

The phone rang loudly beside his bed, jarring him from a deep sleep. Groping for it with his eyes still closed, Jake found the receiver and brought it gingerly to his ear.

"Ugh... um, yes?"

"Jake? Are you up yet?"

"Um, no, Sal, not quite. I must have dozed off again after the alarm went off," said Jake, glancing over at his clock radio. He groaned. It was 10:30 and he felt terrible. Thank God it was Saturday. It *was* Saturday, wasn't it? He felt a momentary panic at the prospect of having to go in to work feeling like this.

"How are you feeling?" said Sally. "Any better?"

"Well, it's all relative, I suppose," said Jake, rubbing his temples. "I'm alive, I can still feel all my limbs and my eyes are working—just about."

Sally laughed. "Well," she said, "I've got plans for today. How about a nice hike, followed by a light dinner at my place? A little exercise might help you work this out of your system."

"Believe me, it's already worked its way out of my system," Jake said, looking around as if to find an excuse. He caught sight of himself in the mirror on his dresser and leaned over to get a better look. His hair was disheveled, he had dark rings under his eyes and his lips were dry and cracked. Not a pretty sight.

"Sal, I'd better pass on today," he said, thinking that a day in bed was more what he had in mind.

"Jake, how can you waste a perfectly good Saturday?" said Sally. "You'll feel fine as soon as you get up and move around. Look, I'll bring you over some supplements and some other stuff to perk you up and you'll be ready to go by lunchtime. How's that sound?"

Bloody awful, thought Jake, wishing he hadn't given her a

key. "Sweetheart, I appreciate your concern and you going to all that trouble, but really I'd rather just lie low today," he said. "I wouldn't be good company anyway, so you'd be far better off spending the day on your own."

"That's pathetic," said Sally. "You'll have to come up with something better than that. I wouldn't dream of leaving you to suffer on your own on a beautiful day like this. I'll be there in half an hour." She hung up, and Jake fell back against the pillows, too exhausted to argue.

He eased himself into a sitting position, got slowly out of bed and headed for the bathroom. His head was pounding, his tongue felt furry and his insides were raw and tender. What the hell had he eaten last night? He couldn't even remember. As soon as he did, though, he would make a mental note to never eat whatever-it-was again.

He took a shower, standing under the hot needles of water in the hope that it would revive him and clear his foggy brain. He dried himself slowly. His whole body felt fragile and shaky. He must be getting old, he thought. Eating out never affected him like this before. Rubbing foam on his chin, he was just about to start shaving when the doorbell rang. He groaned. That was a quick half-hour, he thought.

"Jake, it's me," called Sally, letting herself in. "Take your time getting ready. I'll just fix you something special while I'm waiting."

He heard her walk across the hall and into the kitchen. Resuming his shaving, he wondered what she had in store for him. Bound to be some healthy stuff, he thought. Probably snake oil mixed with raw egg yolks and goat's whey protein powder with some of that awful green stuff she took every morning. His stomach churned at the thought.

He dried his chins, combed his hair and decided that he looked almost presentable. Returning to the bedroom, he pulled on some shorts and a T-shirt, and padded barefoot down the stairs.

Sally was in the living room, curled up on the leather couch.

She smiled at him as he came in, and got up to give him a hug. "Jake, you look terrible," she said, stepping back to look at him.

"Thanks," he said. "I think I'll just make some coffee to wake me up." He turned towards the kitchen. "Want some?"

"No," said Sally, following him into the kitchen. "It's probably the worst thing you could possibly have, after what you've been through."

"What I've been through *was* the worst thing," said Jake, irritated. "Things can only get better." He reached for the coffeepot but Sally took his arm and pulled him round to face her.

"Jake, sweetie, it will only aggravate and stimulate your system—which is already exhausted. You need something to restore you, not whip you into overtime. I've got just the thing to soothe your nerves, calm your stomach and get rid of that headache."

"How'd you know I had a headache?" said Jake, grudgingly.

"I'm psychic," she said, smiling. "Now drink this." She held up a large glass of thick, pale-green liquid.

*I knew it,* thought Jake. *It's that awful green stuff.* "What's in it?" he said suspiciously. "It looks like it came from that pond in your back garden."

She laughed, and led him back into the living room. "It's nothing but goodness," she said. "Now I know that's a scary prospect because you're not used to it, but it might actually make you feel human again."

"You still haven't told me what's in it," he said, taking the glass from her and sniffing the contents.

"It's a combination of protein powder, fresh papaya, blue green algae—"

"It *is* from your pond!" said Jake, hurriedly putting the glass down on the coffee table as if he'd just had a close brush with death. "I'm not drinking this stuff. What are you trying to do to me, woman?"

"Calm down, Jake," said Sally soothingly. "It's not from my pond. It's a very potent, nutritious food that's harvested from pristine lakes. It's full of minerals, protein, chlorophyll—"

"That stuff's fine for plants," said Jake. "You can't expect me to drink it. What's it supposed to do to me, anyway?"

"It will help clean out your liver, for starters," said Sally, picking up the glass and putting it back in his hand. "It will also give your system lots of good enzymes to fight bacteria, as well as providing protein to rebuild all those damaged cells and transport all those important trace minerals."

"What makes you think I need all this?" said Jake, still suspicious.

"One look at you would be enough to convince an entire jury—beyond a shadow of a doubt," Sally laughed. "Now why on earth would you have such resistance to feeling better?"

"I don't. I'm just worried it might do me in. Okay, okay," he said, raising his hands to fend off her next protest, "I'll try it." He lifted the glass to his lips and took a sip.

"Careful!" said Sally. "You don't want to overdo it."

"Very funny," said Jake, taking another sip. "It's not too bad, I suppose, considering…"

"Good," said Sally. "Drink up and we'll get going."

"It's not *that* good, Sal," said Jake. "I'm still in serious condition and a hike might do me more harm than good."

"I doubt it," said Sally, leaning over to massage his temples. "Why don't you just lie back on the couch and I'll give you a massage…"

"Great," said Jake, putting down the glass and turning over onto his stomach.

"…before we go," Sally finished.

He groaned but said nothing as she began to knead his shoulders.

"Just relax," said Sally, taking some oil from her bag beside the couch. "This will help relieve the tension in your muscles." She poured some yellow liquid into the palm of her hand and rubbed both hands together vigorously before resuming her massage. A pungent aroma filled Jake's nostrils and he sighed in contentment.

"Whassat?" he asked, out of the side of his mouth.

"My own special blend of bergamot, patchouli, geranium and lavender oils," said Sally.

"Mmmm," said Jake, feeling his insides finally begin to subside. "I just might get sick more often."

"I wouldn't recommend it," said Sally. "Next time, it'll be castor oil and coffee enemas."

# 7
# Liver enlightenment

"Ohmmmmm... Ohhmmmm…" Sitting cross-legged, leaning against the wall on one side of the vast liver chamber, with his hands resting on his knees and his eyes closed, Jeremy Gene was meditating. As he continued to chant the ancient mantra, he began to feel a profound lightness and peace descend upon him. *I really ought to do this more often*, he thought, then realized his mind was wandering and forced himself to concentrate once again on the mantra.

"Ohhhmmmm," he intoned, feeling the sound vibrate up through his head. "Ohh…" he stopped, a grating sound breaking his concentration. He opened one eye and found himself face to face with a bright green figure that looked like an alien from another planet.

"Who the hell are you?" he asked, irritated at having his serenity disrupted.

"Name's Phyll," said the stranger, "Chloro Phyll, actually." Jeremy saw that he was holding the nozzle of some contraption that he had been pulling along the ground behind him—obviously the source of the grating sound.

"Don't you have any respect?" said Jeremy, glowering at him. "Don't you know that this place—" he gestures around the liver chamber, "—is the seat of intuition?"

"Well, it sounds more like the seat of anger to me," said Phyll. "What were you doing, anyway? Sounded as if you were in pain."

"I was meditating!" said Jeremy indignantly. "Are you from another galaxy or what?"

"Now that you mention it, I am feeling rather alienated," said Phyll. "Normally I'm greeted with open arms because I go around cleaning up messes."

"That's great, Phyll, but you wrecked my concentration."

"Well, don't mind me," said Phyll. "You just carry on with what you're doing and I'll just do my vacuuming." He leaned down and flicked a switch on his machine, filling the chamber with a noise like a lawnmower.

"How do you expect me to meditate with you making all that noise?" shouted Jeremy, exasperated.

"Well, wait till I'm finished, then," Phyll shouted back over his shoulder.

"When will that be?" asked Jeremy.

"Could be two or three years, depending on whether I get back-up or not."

"Two or three ye—! Now wait a minute," said Jeremy, hurrying after him, all serenity long gone. "Turn that thing off for a second, would you."

"Sorry, can't hear you," shouted Phyll, his back to him.

"I said turn it off!" roared Jeremy.

"Definitely the seat of anger," said Phyll calmly, reaching down to turn off the machine.

"Whose orders are you acting on?" said Jeremy. "I've never seen you in here before. Are you sure you're in the right place?"

"So much for intuition," said Phyll. "Yeah, I'm in the right place. Her majesty over there gave the orders herself." Phyll gestured with his thumb in the direction of the glass-fronted office at the other end of the chamber. Inside, Jeremy could see Lily Liver sitting at her desk, her glasses perched halfway down her nose as she wrote furiously on the pad in front of her.

"Well, we'll see about this," he said, bristling with anger as he marched off down the corridor.

Lily Liver looked up as he came in. "Hold it right there," she said, putting up her hand. "I know what you're going to say and there's nothing I can do about it."

"But I can't meditate with this going on," said Jeremy, gesturing behind him. "Is nothing sacred any more?"

"You think you've got it bad?" said Lily, taking off her glasses and peering at him sternly. "I've got over 500 different functions to perform down here, and look at this backlog." She tapped the stacks of paper on the desk and gestured to more piles on the floor. "I've got to coordinate crews to deal with preservatives, colourings, all kinds of toxins, hormones, cholesterol, and sugar levels, not to mention filtering out the blood and keeping everyone in a good mood. This clean-up job is top priority, so I'm afraid that your meditating will have to wait, Jeremy. Any other questions?"

"Em, I don't know," said Jeremy, somewhat chastened. "Well, actually, yes, there is one," he said, turning as he reached the door. "Isn't meditating just as beneficial? I mean, what if we all did it and went on a fast or something; wouldn't that help?"

"Jeremy, there's no point in sitting there contemplating your navel if you're up to your ears in junk food and toxic debris," said Lily patiently. "And fasting only weakens everyone, depriving them of the strength they would need to clean up this mess. First, the body has to be fed some potent nutrients so that it is strong enough to get rid of this stuff; then it has to be cleaned up. Only after all that can you start to effectively use the mind to reach higher states of being. If you try to meditate while the body is in such a state of degeneration, you'll end up being ungrounded and scattered all over the place."

"I see," said Jeremy. "So I've got a long wait ahead of me before I can be enlightened."

"Well, that all depends on His Lordship," said Lily. "If he sends down more of this good stuff on a regular basis, and eliminates the junk food, alcohol and cigarettes, there's a chance that you could resume your practice in about six months' time."

"Now I'm depressed. I don't know what to do with myself."

"Well, you can help me sort through this lot, for starters," said Lily, handing him a pen and indicating the chair on the other side of the desk. "None of us is going to feel any better until this backlog is cleared. It's clogging up the entire system and things are starting to malfunction."

Jeremy looked down at the heaps of paper, and then over his shoulder at Phyll busily vacuuming. Sighing heavily, he pulled out the chair and sat down.

"Here," said Lily, passing him a folder. "I have a union meeting at 10:30 tonight, so this will be a great help." She stood up, putting some papers into her briefcase.

"Why so late?" asked Jeremy.

"It's the only time most of the staff is off duty," said Lily. "His Lordship finally gives everyone a rest by about 10pm—except for you, of course."

"Me? What do you mean?"

"Well, I'm putting you in charge of the reproductive department so you'll probably only start to get busy around that time. According to the latest bulletin from Command Central, there should be some activity in that area this evening. Think you can handle that?"

"No!" said Jeremy, alarmed. "I've never done this before."

"Don't worry," said Lily with a dismissive wave of her hand as she headed out the door. "Just use your intuition."

# 8
# Active resistance

"I can't climb that!" said Jake in horror as he squinted up at the mountain. "I can't even see the top."

"Well, that's only because you're still at the bottom," said Sally cheerfully. "Anyway, we don't have to go all the way to the top—just as far as your virile, muscle-bound body can take you. Come on, Jake, you'll feel great afterwards."

"Sal, darling, see this trail here down along the river," said Jake pointing to his right. "Couldn't we start off with that and—"

"Nah, that's for wimps," said Sally, hoisting her knapsack onto her back. "Now let's just check that we have enough water before we get going. We don't want you getting dehydrated again."

"It's not water I need to worry about," said Jake. "More like a stretcher, smelling salts and a cable car. A man in my condition—"

"You used to love this," Sally interrupted him, taking him by the arm as they started off on the trail. "Do you remember when we first met and used to spend all weekend hiking?"

"Course I do," said Jake. "And it was fun. But I was fit then, Sal. I've had a lot of stress at work since then and I just haven't had the energy or time to do this stuff."

"But that was only nine months ago," said Sally. "Surely you can't have lost all that vitality in that short time?"

"Well, no, of course I haven't," said Jake somewhat doubtfully. "It's all still in there, somewhere." He grinned, poking his full stomach, then turned to face her.

"What are you, anyway—witch or woman?"

Sally laughed. "Oh, probably a bit of both. Look," she said, pointing to the bushes alongside the trail. "Blackberries. We can nibble as we go."

"Allow me, madam," said Jake, reaching up to pick some of the large, black berries swollen from the recent rain.

"Thanks, Galahad," said Sally as he popped two berries into her mouth. "Did you know that blackberries are rich in vitamin C but also contain a lectin that aggravates your digestive system—if you have blood type O?"

"No, I didn't," said Jake. "But now, finally, I feel complete. I always knew there was something missing in my life and now I've found it. How can I ever repay you?" He looked at her earnestly.

Sally laughed, and punched him in the shoulder. 'You're always teasing me," she said. "You know, I miss being out in nature together—like this." She breathed deeply, and gestured with her arm at the blue sky, the trees and the mountain before them. "And I hate to see you unwell."

"I'm fine, Sal, really," said Jake, taking her hand again as they continued along the trail. "I'm just overworked at the office. Once things quieten down, I'll get out and about more."

"Well, I hope so," said Sally, doubtfully. "I'm not too keen on short-term investments."

"I'll outlive you, woman," said Jake. "Come back and see me in your next incarnation. Okay, so I may be just a little overweight. But, I have to admit, I am beginning to feel a little more energetic after that magic potion of yours."

"Well that's good," said Sally. "It usually feels good, at first."

"What do you mean, 'at first'?" said Jake, beginning to breathe heavily as the trail steepened.

"If the body has a backlog of toxins to clean out and other repairs to do, as soon as it starts to build enough strength and get all the nutrients it needs, it goes to work. Initially, you feel good because it gives you a boost of goodness. But then that goodness is taken to where it's most needed, and all other unnecessary activities are curtailed."

"What does that mean?" said Jake, looking worried.

"It means a period of detoxification, during which you have to take things easy," said Sally. "Usually, you feel extremely tired and grouchy, because the body is doing all it can to take the toxins out of your tissues, and into the blood stream so that they can be eliminated. It's a lot of hard work, and the body needs all the help it can get in order to do it. That means that anything you do to hinder that process, such as drinking, smoking, over-exerting yourself or eating unhealthy foods, will make it extremely difficult—if not impossible—for the body to heal itself."

"Sounds like I'll need lots of time in bed," said Jake, grinning at her. They climbed in silence for a while, Sally setting a steady pace with Jake stopping every so often to catch his breath.

"What if I don't do this?" said Jake, stopping. "You're the one with all the nutritional training. What's the prognosis, Doc?"

"Well, if you really want to know, you'll probably develop some kind of degenerative disease in your mid-to-late forties," said Sally, reaching into her pack for her water bottle. "The body can only cope with so much, you know, and then it starts to break down. You hear about people waking up one morning with cancer, but it doesn't happen like that. It develops slowly over time, sneaking up on you without you realizing it."

"Bit like you, really," said Jake, grinning. He pulled her into a bear hug and kissed her full on the lips. "You look beautiful, Sal, with your hair all lit up by the sun, colour in your cheeks, and little ladylike beads of sweat trickling down your neck, right here. I wonder where they go." He leaned over to peer down her shirt, and Sally laughed, taking his hand again and resuming the climb.

"I, on the other hand," Jake continued, "am the quintessential Cliffhanger type—hairy chest covered in beads of macho sweat, calf muscles bulging with every step, and—"

"...great heaving gasps for breath," Sally finished with a smile. "Yup, very manly."

# 9
# Into the HeartHand

Arnie Aorta was sweating profusely. He hadn't had a workout like this in ages. "What the heck is His Lordship up to today?" he said to Heather Heart as he worked the aortic valve. "His pulse must be up over 150."

"According to E&E, he's climbing a mountain," said Heather, consulting the monitor in front of her. "His pulse is 145 and his blood pressure is also high. Watch that flow there, Arnie, it's looking a little irregular."

"I know, I know," said Arnie, wiping the sweat from his brow. "But I'm having a hard time keeping up with him. I've only been working half-time for the past four months and I'm out of practice."

"Well I think Lawrence is having an even harder time of it," said Heather. "I should give him a call to see how he's doing." She reached for her cell phone and dialed the 5864 (LUNG) extension.

"Lawrence Lung here. This had better be good."

"Lawrence, it's Heather. Just wondered how you're doing over there."

"Heather, we're so busy, I'm not taking calls from anyone but you," said Lawrence, sounding flustered. "We're churning out that oxygenated blood just as fast as you pump the deoxygenated stuff in here. But we're having a hell of a time with all that nicotine and God knows how many chemicals from those fags His Lordship smokes. We could work twice as fast and efficiently without that clogging up the works. You should see the wallpaper down here—just covered in black marks. Disgusting. Doesn't look like we'll ever get it redone. It used to be a nice delicate shade of pink and now it's—"

"Yes, Lawrence, I know. Well, I mustn't keep you," said

Heather. "Just wanted to check if there was anything we could do to help at this end."

"Just keep on pumping that stuff over here," said Lawrence. "Actually, it's not coming through as powerfully as it should. Is there some weakness in the system over there?"

"Well, the muscle is in poor shape because it hasn't been used like this for a while," said Heather. "We've also had to cope with a lot of fatty deposits building up in the main arteries, so traffic has been slow and there's been a lot of congestion. Arthur Artery should be arriving shortly to do some clean-up and traffic control down south. Should reduce some of the pressure."

"Who's Arthur Artery?" said Lawrence.

"He's a new guy who arrived yesterday. He's a traffic engineer who specializes in arterial flow but he's also done some work in weather forecasting so he should be able to help us predict climatic changes sooner. He's been asked to do a full survey of the organism and to submit a report to CC."

"If only we could get some more unpolluted air down here," said Lawrence, sounding distracted. "Do you have any idea what happens to my crew when His Lordship has a coughing fit? We had tornado conditions here last week after that dairy overdose, and half the guys went on strike. And the mucous! Can't he tell that it's causing a problem? And if he could start taking vitamins E and C as well as some CoQ10 to enhance the oxygen supply, we'd all be a lot better off. Not to mention lipotropic factors for reducing the fat content of the blood. That would help with your problem, too, Heather, and—"

"Why don't you bring it up at the meeting later, Lawrence," said Heather. "I must go. My other line is ringing. Keep up the good work." She hung up, took a deep breath, then picked up the other line.

"Heather Heart. How can I help you?"

"Heather, this is Arthur. I'm on my way but I think I'm going to need directions. It's like spaghetti junction down here and I haven't a clue where I'm going."

"Right," said Heather, moving back in front of her monitor.

"Where exactly are you now, Arthur?"

"Well I'm heading west on the main artery. Is that right?"

"Yes," said Heather. "Now you need to look out for exit 160, marked Vena Cava. Take that turn-off heading south and—"

"Just a minute, Heather. I think I'm going to need to write this down," said Arthur. "Hold on till I find my pen... Okay, go ahead."

"Once you come off at the Vena Cava exit, you'll see signs for Skittish Airways as you pass through Lung Labyrinth. Keep on going, following the red signs for Vena Cava until you reach the Heartland. Once you get there, follow the signs for the Heart Centre, and you can park anywhere outside the Right Ventricle building. I'll be inside at the main console. It's busy on the highways right now, so you may encounter some congestion, but do your best."

"I'll just go with the flow," said Arthur.

Heather hung up and turned back to her monitor. "You can probably ease up for a few seconds, Arnie. Looks like some warm and fuzzy feelings coming down. Pulse is slowing and blood pressure has dropped. Won't last long, though. His Lordship is still only halfway up the mountain, according to the last E&E-mail."

"Oh, heck," said Arnie, gasping for breath. "What's it going to take to get his Lordship back on the straight and narrow?"

"A miracle," said Heather, shaking her head.

# 10
# Strategy and subterfuge

"Order, please, order," said Brian Brain, tapping his spoon against his glass. The buzz of conversation subsided and he looked around the table to check for absentees. All 20 chairs were occupied. "Looks as if all the department heads are here, with Oliver standing in for Lily. Glad you could join us, Oliver." Oliver grunts in acknowledgement but doesn't look up. "Right, let's get started." Brian turns to Crystal, seated on his right. "You've got the agenda, Crystal, so go ahead, please."

"Well, we all know that there's been some upheaval lately," Crystal said, standing up. There were murmurs of agreement and a general nodding of heads. "And we've got several departments in a crisis situation. We need to know exactly what is required in these areas so that we can submit requisitions for what we need. Oliver, why don't you go first since you seem eager to speak." She gestured towards Oliver who was fidgeting in his seat and tapping his pen impatiently on his pad.

"Too right," said Oliver, jumping to his feet. "I don't know how much more of this I can take. I would like a direct missive to be sent to His Lordship so that he understands the gravity of the situation down here. Lily and I have had an inhuman backlog to cope with lately and this has got to stop!"

"Okay, Oliver, take it easy," said Brian. "Just tell us exactly what's going on."

"I can't take it easy; that's the problem," said Oliver, distraught. "My job is to filter off toxins from normal, everyday stuff designed to nourish His Lordship and keep things running relatively smoothly. I can cope with the odd over-indulgence, no problem. But I refuse to act as the fall guy for the whimsical sugar cravings of his spoilt palate and stomach, which, for some reason, seem to think they rule the roost down here."

"Now, hold on there just a minute," said Sam Stomach indignantly, getting to his feet.

"It's okay, Sam," said Brian, motioning him back into his seat. "I think Oliver just needs to vent a bit."

"If I decide to stop clearing garbage out of the system, then you're all toast," Oliver waved his arm around the table. "What do you think happens when his Lordship sends down a shitload of sugary stuff at midnight, sending the whole crew into heavy-duty overtime, and then he buggers off to sleep?"

"Oliver, please, watch your language," said Crystal, embarrassed.

"Well, I'll tell you what happens," Oliver continued, oblivious to the reprimand. "We end up working an all-nighter, which would be fine, if we didn't have to work during the day or if we could take some time off. And, to make matters worse, when his Lordship drifts off to slumberland, all our usual energy systems get shut down so that we have to work with a skeleton crew. And then I get flack from everyone else. I have Sophie venting her spleen, Billy Gallbladder getting bilious, not to mention Karl and Kyla Kidney complaining about all the peeing caused by so much stress. There have been so many toxins coming our way from Colon County that fat is starting to build up in the blood, sugar levels are going haywire, and even the hormones are getting out of hand. I can't be responsible for the consequences, but it will be interesting to see how good His Lordship is at liver repair. Not quite as easy as fixing the lawnmower, you know." He stopped, breathing heavily, and looked around the table, as if seeing the others for the first time. "We have to do something, Brian," he said quietly. "This is serious."

"We get your point, Oliver," said Brian. "What do you suggest we do? We've already put numerous requisitions through the system but they don't seem to be getting through."

"We have to give him a scare, then," said Oliver, "something to get his attention so that he realizes what's happening down here."

The others exchanged nervous glances, murmuring among themselves.

"Quiet, please," said Brian. "What exactly had you in mind, Oliver?"

"Well, ultimately we want to get him to improve his diet and digestion, which will benefit us all and prevent the entire system from crashing. But for now, I suggest a severe low-blood-sugar attack—something to put him on his back so that he's forced to stop and think about what he's doing."

"But then we get the blame," said Pete Pancreas, indignant. "Everyone thinks that we're the only ones responsible for the blood sugar levels and they don't realize that we work together."

"It's not important what anyone thinks," said Oliver. "We just want to scare him into taking some positive action."

"Okay," said Brian. "If we decide to do this—and we'll take a vote in a minute—how exactly would we do it?"

"I've got it all worked out," said Oliver, reaching into his briefcase. "I've typed up some instructions that we will all need to read and follow to the letter." He began passing out sheets of paper to the others. There were more murmurs as they began to read.

"What happens if some serious damage is done?" said Heather. "How do we know this won't get out of hand?"

"Crystal can monitor everything at Command," said Oliver. "Please explain, Crystal."

Crystal glanced at the sheet once again before standing up. "Oliver's right. We can keep a close watch on things from upstairs. I can monitor blood-sugar levels, pulse, blood pressure, temperature, etc, and if anything looks dicey, we should be able to make adjustments to compensate. There's always a risk, of course, but if what Oliver says is true, then it's worth it. We could be in for something much more serious if we don't take some immediate action."

"If sugar levels in the blood get dangerously low, we can bring in some hormones to help Lily and Oliver download some of that stored glycogen from the liver into the blood," said Andrew Adrenal. "If, by any chance, there's too much glucose in the blood, we'll have you standing by, Pete, ready to let Lily and Oliver know so that they can bring in more insulin to remove some of that glucose. It's a matter of fine-tuning and we'll have to stay in constant contact by cell phone."

"Okay," said Brian. "Sounds as if it could work. Any other questions?"

"What kind of hormones will you need to have on hand?" asked Oliver.

"Stand by with cortisone, adrenaline and corticosteroids, just in case," said Crystal. "You'll have to check with Andrew and Pat to see when they need them."

"I'll probably need to produce some more corticotropin too," said Pat Pituitary, "so that I can support you, Andy. Just let me know if you need any help."

"So when do we do this?" said Brian, anxious to conclude the matter.

"Mid-morning tomorrow," said Oliver. "That's when His Lordship tends to do the most damage. He starts the day with coffee or just has a sweet, sticky bun, which sends us all into hyperactivity. Then, at around 11am, his energy systems crash. That's the time to do it."

"Wait," said Crystal, sifting through the pile of notes in front of her. "I've got a better idea. His Lordship is making an important presentation to some clients tomorrow at midday. He's launching a new advertising campaign that he's just developed, and it's extremely important to him."

"Isn't that being a bit too hard on him" said Heather. "I mean, we don't want him getting depressed and even more stressed."

"Look, we can't have you going all soft-hearted and sentimental on us, Heather," said Oliver. "This is the survival of the entire organism we're talking about here. If it goes down, so do all of us. He's got to be made to see the vital importance of doing something about it. If we just stage it at home, with nobody there to witness it, he won't take it so seriously."

"Actually," Lily intervened, "I think the matter may already be taken care of."

"What do you mean, Lily?" asked Brian, as all eyes turned towards her.

"Well, I just put Jeremy in charge of the Erectile Console, in the reproductive department," said Lily, smiling. "He's got absolutely no experience in that area and I'm sure there'll be a few, eh, cock-ups, to say the least. Normally, there's an efficient, competent team on duty down there, and his Lordship is not used to things not working smoothly. I'm sure he'll think it's to do with his health and start worrying. "

"I don't think it's enough," said Oliver. "He might just pass it off as fatigue after that strenuous hike. I still think we should go with my plan."

"Well, let's take a vote on it, then," said Brian briskly. "How many in favour of Oliver's proposal?" He looked around the table as the others thought for a moment. Then, slowly, hands began to go up. Heather remained doubtful, looking around her uncertainly as her colleagues voted in favour. "That makes 17 for, and one against, not counting Crystal and me," said Brian. "That's already a large majority in favour, so let's do it."

"There *is* a God," said Oliver, looking relieved.

"Okay, meeting's adjourned," said Brian. "I know some of you have to get back to your stations so we'll cover the rest of the agenda next week. If anything urgent comes up before tomorrow morning, contact either Crystal or me." He looked around the table again, his expression earnest. "Good luck, everyone. Let's not screw this one up. It may be the only chance we get."

# 11
# A quickie

"Thank God," said Jake, as he slumped onto Sally's couch. "I survived yet another grueling challenge by the indomitable, slave-driving Miss Sally. Never let it be said that life with you is boring, Sal. On the contrary; it's all the more precious because you never know if you're going to survive from one minute to the next."

"Jake, you exaggerate," said Sally, pulling off her boots. "You loved every minute of it, once you got into a rhythm."

"I got into arrhythmia, no problem," said Jake. "I just hope I can get out of it." He grinned at her, enjoying their easy banter and her ready smile. "Sal, let's just go to bed, have dinner later." He twirled her round to face him and kissed her passionately on the lips. She started to object so he kissed her again. "No buts. Dinner will keep. You're coming upstairs with me."

# 12
# Penile servitude

Jeremy was staring at the controls on the Penis Panel, scratching his head. There were so many different levers and lights that he had no idea where to start. "Teddy, can't you help me with this?" he said, frustrated. "Nope," said Teddy Testosterone, who was lounging in a chair by the fire, clipping his nails. "I don't know the first thing about that stuff. All I know is that when that there red light goes on, I go into action. Till then, I'm off duty."

"Well, thanks a lot," said Jeremy. "Don't expect any help from me if things get hectic later on. Once I get these levers worked out, I'm out of here. You'll be on your own."

"Used to it," said Teddy nonchalantly, examining his manicure. "There's a manual under the shelf that might help."

"Why didn't you tell me that sooner?" Jeremy glared at him, reaching down for the thick red binder on the floor beside his feet. "This is huge. How on earth can there be so much information on just one tiny area?"

"It's a complex organism," said Teddy. "And His Lordship wouldn't be too happy to hear you calling it tiny. There's an awful lot more to it than most people think."

"Oh," said Jeremy, leafing through the manual. "I thought it was just a simple matter of operating these levers at the right time, and that was it. This green one here must be the 'ON' lever and this red one is obviously 'OFF.' But they're both in the inactive position. I don't get it. And what's this other one, here, that seems to be active right now?" He pointed to a blue lever, to the right of the panel.

"Oh that's 'Lever Alone,'" said Teddy, grinning. "That's a sort of stand-by lever for when it might be unwise for his Lordship to make any advances, but he's still hopeful. It helps to keep his mind elsewhere until the timing is right."

"Sooo," said Jeremy, absorbed in the manual. "The green lever is to turn him on, and the red one is to turn him off. Got that. And when the red light comes on, what exactly do *you* do?"

"Well, I stoke this fire here and add plenty of fuel to it to really get it going. Then I sit back and watch the action."

"What action?" said Jeremy.

"See this pleasure gauge here?" said Teddy, pointing to a dial on the console in front of Jeremy. "When that reaches its maximum level, you have to turn on that green lever."

"Well, that's easy enough," said Jeremy, visibly relieved.

"Yeah, that part is. But then you have to be able to hold it in place, which takes a fair bit of muscle. And, at the crucial moment, you have to press this auto-eject button here," he pointed to a large arrow-shaped button on the console, "which will release the pressure. You also need to know when to let go of the green lever and engage the red one. It's a matter of very delicate timing. And if you get it wrong, well..."

"Well what? What could happen?"

"You could get yourself into serious trouble with Edgar Ego."

"I've heard about him, but I've never met him," said Jeremy. "He has no idea who *I* am, though."

"That won't matter," said Teddy. "He gets around and he'll find you if he wants to."

"I've heard that he can be quite nasty," said Jeremy, worried again.

"Nasty?" said Teddy sarcastically. "Hell hath no fury like Edgar's. He's in charge of the corporate image and if he's made to look like a fool, he shows no mercy."

"But what could he do to me?"

"Mmmm, let's see," said Teddy thoughtfully, scratching his head. "Well, the last time something happened in this neck of the woods was about ten years ago, when His Lordship was a lot younger. A student of Lily's was on duty at the time and he screwed up. He got the levers and timing all wrong and it was a mess. Edgar was down here so fast the poor guy hardly had time to say 'Ooops'. He was disgraced and ridiculed at a staff meeting in front of everyone and Edgar made sure he was out of work for several months."

"Well, that's not too bad, really," said Jeremy, considering the situation.

"Then," said Teddy, continuing, "he was condemned to working in the archives, and you know how mind-numbing that is. The poor bugger never got ahead after that. Still, I'm sure that will never happen to you. Better keep an eye on that gauge, though."

"Huh? Oh, crikey," said Jeremy, hurriedly turning back to the console. "The temperature's rising, Teddy. Remind me what to do again..."

"Sorry, can't right now," said Teddy. "Got to focus on this fire." He began stoking the embers, throwing on some logs from the basket beside him.

"But it's climbing so rapidly," said Jeremy, panicking. "It's almost at the maximum point." *Stay calm*, he told himself. *Use your intuition*, Lily had said. If he could just get a feel for it, he'd do fine. He took hold of the green lever with his right hand and closed his eyes. Concentrating hard, he tried to tune into what was happening.

★ ★ ★

Sally lay naked on her back, nestled in the thick flowery quilt on her bed. Leaning over her, Jake was kissing her tenderly all over, making her moan with pleasure. His hands followed the curves of her body, and his fingers ran through her hair.

"Sal, you're so beautiful," he said, his voice husky. "I want to make love to you all night long."

Sally murmured in response and kissed him deeply on the lips. Then, pushing him gently off her, she rolled over onto her side and began sensually caressing him. After a few minutes, Jake grabbed her hand, breathing hard. "God, woman, look what you do to me," he said. He rolled on top of her again and reached between her legs.

★ ★ ★

The sweat was running down Jeremy's face as the pleasure gauge hit maximum. Gritting his teeth, he pulled down hard on the green lever with both hands, throwing all his weight behind it to hold it in place. He could feel it vibrating, almost as if it were alive, and he closed his eyes again to better focus on the task. Shouldn't have to hold on too long, he told himself. No one could maintain this kind of pressure. A bead of sweat trickled into his eye and he wiped it away with his left hand. As he did so, his right hand, slippery from all the perspiration, slipped off the lever, releasing it back into the 'off' position. *Oh, no,* thought Jeremy. *I've done it now.*

★ ★ ★

"Jake, honey, what's wrong?" asked Sally, concerned. "Are you too tired?"

"No," said Jake, bewildered. "I... it's never happened before. I don't know what's going on."

"It's okay, sweetheart," said Sally soothingly. "You've probably overdone it today. Don't worry about it."

"No, no, it can't be that," Jake said. "Just a momentary blip, that's all. There, see?"

★ ★ ★

Jeremy grabbed the green lever again, pulling it back down into the ON position. He could feel the pressure behind it and, despite the sweat trickling down his forehead, he held on grimly with both hands. *What's the crucial point?* he wondered. *How do I know when to push that eject button?* He looked at the console, hoping for some inspiration, but found none. The needle on the pleasure gauge was still hovering around maximum and showed no signs of dropping. Exhausted, Jeremy decided it was time to make an executive decision.

★ ★ ★

Jake was perspiring heavily, his breathing shallow and rapid. He positioned himself above Sally, about to enter her, when suddenly he froze. He looked down at himself in horror and rolled onto his back with a loud moan.

★ ★ ★

*Phew!* Jeremy flopped back in his chair. *I think I timed it just right.* He wiped the sweat off his brow and sat back in his chair. "What do you think, Teddy?" He turned to see Teddy slumped over the arm of his chair, fast asleep. Jeremy pushed his chair over to Teddy and shook him vigorously. "Teddy! Wake up. I've finished, and I need to know what to do next."

"I'd get the hell out of here, if I were you," said Teddy, glancing at the console where Jeremy had been working. "I think that was a bit premature. Won't be long before Edgar makes his presence felt."

# 13
## Domestic showdown

"Jake, it's okay, honey. Don't worry. It was a long hike and you're probably still recovering from yesterday. It's no big deal."

"Yeah." Jake lay on his back, staring at the ceiling.

"Come on, let's get dinner. I'm ravenous. We can curl up on the couch afterwards and maybe watch a film." She leaned over and kissed him on the cheek.

"Okay." He smiled half-heartedly and watched her pull on a long baggy T-shirt. She reached out her hand. He hesitated for a moment then took her hand and eased himself out of bed. He slipped on his shorts and followed her downstairs to the kitchen.

"Sit and I'll get everything ready," said Sally, gesturing towards a kitchen chair. "There's chicken and spinach salad, with poppy seed vinaigrette, and sourdough whole grain bread, followed by homemade blackberry crumble."

"After all you said about blackberries!" said Jake, taking a seat at the table.

"Well, I'm fairly sure you're not blood type O, so don't worry," said Sally, laughing. "If you were, you would be like our early ancestors—a lean, mean predator type, always active and on the look-out for prey."

"Are you blind, woman? 'Course I'm type O. I'm sizing up my prey this very second," said Jake, ogling her intently.

"Aren't you forgetting about the 'lean' part?" said Sally.

"Don't be fooled. It's in there, just temporarily buried," said Jake. He frowned suddenly, slumping over the table as he watched Sally bustling around the kitchen, putting placemats on the table and taking some knives and forks from a small drawer under the countertop.

"I thought we might just stick with water, after the hike," said Sally. "Alcohol might not be a good idea after last night."

"Hell, I'm exhausted," said Jake, dropping his head onto the table.

"That's normal, after all we've done today, Jake," said Sally, soothingly, moving towards him.

"It's not from the hike, Sal. It's this. Us." He gestured around the room, stopping Sally in her tracks. "I can't take all this pressure. I feel as if I'm going to explode. Nothing I do seems okay with you. Now I can't even perform in bed. I feel controlled, monitored, policed."

"What do you mean," said Sally, stunned, her heart fluttering in a panic.

"You watch every move I make and jump on me if it's not healthy or sensible. I can't make any choices of my own without some kind of fallout."

"You're free to do whatever you want." Sally stood rigidly beside the table, arms folded tightly across her chest. "I'm just making some suggestions because I care for you and you don't seem to know—"

"That's just it!" Jake felt his anger rising. "You think I don't know any better and so you've got to tell me what to do. You don't like me the way I am. Let's face it." He paused, hit by a sudden realization. "I'll never be good enough for you, no matter how much I change."

"Jake, that's not true. I—"

"What do you want from me, Sal?" He turned to face her, his eyes burning.

"I… um…I just want what's best for you, for us. I don't know. I'm sorry…" She turned away, trembling, unable to hold his gaze.

"Well, when you've figured it out, let me know. I need a break from this." He got up, grabbed his keys and jacket, and headed for the door.

"Wait! That's not fair," Sally yelled, her anger flaring as she caught him by the shoulder and swung him round to face her. "If you took care of yourself, I wouldn't have to. It's totally irresponsible the way men do this—you're all in denial about your health, you indulge in everything, with no regard for what happens later on, when things start to go wrong. Who's going to take care of when you end up with emphysema or need to be spoon-fed when you're drooling after a stroke? Why should I care for you if you don't give a damn about your health?"

"You don't have to take care of me and you don't have to love me, either."

"Okay, then, I won't!"

"Fine." Jake strode towards the front door, not looking back.

"What do *you* want from *me*?" Sally yelled after him.

"Maybe I need to think about that, too," said Jake quietly, opening the door and stepping outside. She stared at him as he turned and closed the door softly behind him.

# 14
# Over the edge

"And these figures show the projected sales revenue over the next three years," said Jake, pointing at the flipchart at the front of the room. Putting down his red marker, he returned to his chair, discreetly eyeing his audience in an attempt to gauge their reaction. "As you can see, gentlemen, they are quite impressive."

Six pairs of eyes looked critically back at him. Jake fiddled with his pen, his heart pounding and an uncomfortable sweatiness breaking out under his arms. A jumble of figures swam in his head. Flow charts, budgets, product lines... *What should he say next? How could he convince them? God, this was too much... why did it have to be this hard...?* He felt so very tired...

"What about the timing of the campaign launch?" asked the marketing director of Vital Foods, currently Jake's most promising and lucrative account. "Should we wait till summer, or will this work just as well for spring?"

"Well," said Jake, jumping up from his seat, and turning to the flipchart again. "I've outlined what I consider to be the most... eh...ideal time frame..." He paused, wiping perspiration from his forehead as a wave of nausea suddenly swept over him. "As you can see..." He reached forward to turn to the next chart, but suddenly his chest contracted with a fierce pain and he couldn't breathe. The room swayed and the ground seemed to be coming up to meet him. He barely had time to groan in dismay as he slid to the floor, clasping his chest and pulling the flipchart down with him.

★ ★ ★

"All systems Red Alert," said Crystal smartly into the PA system. "The organism is down. We need maximum manpower at the adrenal cortex, and emergency remedial action at the Heart Centre. Report back as soon as the organism has been stabilized."

She turned to study her monitor, checking the data currently being transmitted by Heather Heart, Lily Liver and Lawrence Lung. Liver function seemed normal, lung activity appeared to be sluggish but holding its own, but the Heart Centre was labouring, with a weak and erratic heartbeat. As Crystal surveyed her monitors, she realized that reception in Command Central had gone haywire, with static and interference on almost all her screens. She clicked on one and zoomed in on the Heart Centre. It was buzzing with activity. "Heather," she said into her mouthpiece, "what's happening down there?"

"Crystal, we're in crisis here!" shouted Heather, her voice shaky. "We should never have gone ahead with this ridiculous plan of Oliver's. It's far more serious than he said it would be, and we could lose everything—"

"Heather, you must stay calm," said Crystal. "If we panic now, we'll have no chance of staying on top of things. What back-up do you need?"

"Back-up will do no good at all," Heather retorted angrily. "The damage is done. There is nothing we can do. We just have to wait and see if outside intervention can stabilize the organism enough to survive this attack."

"Just a minute, Heather. There's a bulletin coming in…" Crystal studied the monitor again as fresh data flooded the screen. "It looks as if this was purely coincidental. An inflamed artery burst, causing a blood clot, which caused an attack. There's nothing you could have done."

"We should have got him to stop smoking years ago," said Heather. "And his cholesterol… Why wasn't something done sooner? This should never have happened. We are all to blame—"

"Heather, calm down! You know that's not true. You know how hard it is to get His Lordship to make positive changes. Unfortunately, it often takes something like this for him to get the message. We'll just have to hope that this will have the desired effect. Now, please…"

"I'm just fed up with always being expected to be forgiving and loving and compassionate towards others, and not letting things get to me. I'm sick of it. How about some compassion for *us*, for a change? Why do we never even get consulted on things—important things like how to stay alive? I need to be able to make decisions for my own department. I mean, it's outrageous that—"

"Heather, I know. I agree with you. You're absolutely right. But let's just try to get over this crisis and then see what can be done to fundamentally change the system. I think we have an opportunity here to make ourselves heard. Okay?"

"I'll believe it when I see it. I must go. I'm needed here. Bye."

She hung up, and Crystal quickly switched her attention to another part of her screen.

"Brian, we need to ensure that some nutritional information gets downloaded from the memory banks so that we can figure out what would help stabilize things. And all that fear-driven adrenaline released into the system needs to be put to good use."

"Right, Crystal," said Brian, coming into focus on the screen. "Fears are running amok in the system, so I'm activating some neurotransmitters to marshal them into order and direct their movements. We need to get them up from the Gut into the Limbic Region to relay their information mentally and to pacify them. We can't let them run riot down there, causing havoc for everyone. Once that's done, we may see some constructive action taking place on the outside." He rubbed his forehead with some consternation. "But there's something else, Crystal."

"Yes, Brian?"

"I'm picking up some unusual activity in the solar plexus area. Not sure what's going on there. Can you check into it?"

"Will do, Brian. I'll get back to you." Crystal clicked on another icon on her desktop and zoomed in on the Solar Plexus Centre. Brilliant yellow swirling light filled the screen. She leaned closer, the glare from the screen lighting up her puzzled expression. "I've never seen anything like it," she said, shaking her head. Punching in more keys, she asked the computer for an analysis of the matter swirling before her. Within seconds, her monitor was filled with data. "Wow," said Crystal. "I think I need some help with this one."

★ ★ ★

"Get that stretcher in here fast," yelled the orderly. "Put him in OR 3. Dr Jenkins is waiting."

Two paramedics flung open the back doors of the ambulance and whipped out the stretcher. Charging through the Emergency entrance, they headed straight for the operating room. Jake lay unconscious on his back, covered in a blanket, with an oxygen mask over his face. An IV drip dangled from a metal brace and was connected to his left arm. The paramedics raced down the hallway, one of them holding on to the metal frame as they ran.

They turned sharply to the right and entered OR 3 where a young male doctor was waiting, wearing a green operating gown, white cotton hat, white mask and white latex gloves.

Beside him stood two nurses, an anesthetist and a young intern.

"Status?" Dr Jenkins barked at the medics.

"We've done CPR, and managed to bring him back within two minutes. Looks like coronary thrombosis. He's on the clot-buster—streptokinase. Barely hanging in there."

Dr Jenkins turned to the anesthetist. "Phillips, get ready to take him under."

★ ★ ★

Jake had no idea where he was. Everything seemed strangely muffled and out of focus. He was floating, disembodied, formless and light as air. How had he got here? And where was everyone? Where were his legs? Where was his body? He couldn't feel anything. There was nothing but a light mistiness all around him.

He turned, moving in slow motion, and realized he was looking down upon a frenzied scene in what seemed to be an operating room. Intrigued, he saw his own body lying on the operating table, a flurry of activity around it. His chest was open and blood was being siphoned in or out (he wasn't sure which) through tubes trailing in all directions. A nurse was staunching the flow with swabs as a surgeon worked feverishly, a small metal instrument in his hand.

★ ★ ★

"Doctor, we've lost him!"

"Get the paddles. We're going to resuscitate. Stand clear, everyone!" Dr Jenkins pressed two paddles to Jake's chest and sent a jolt of electricity through the lifeless body, lifting it off the operating table.

★ ★ ★

Jake felt a wave of dismay wash over him. *My God, I'm dead!* Yet even as he thought this, he realized he was also strangely detached from the whole process. He felt no pain, just a neutral objectivity and fascination as he looked down at his body on the table. It felt very peaceful up here... Did he really want to go back to all that struggle? But what about Sally? She would be heartbroken. He felt a tug, as if some invisible elastic band were pulling him back to earth.

"Still not back, doctor," he heard one of the nurses say and saw the paddles being applied to his chest again.

"Stand clear again. Last time." Everyone waited, holding their breath, then suddenly the heart monitor pinged back to life. The surgeon straightened up and wiped his sleeve across his forehead. "Okay. He's back. Let's get him stabilized and close him up. We've done all we can."

Cradling his bloodied, gloved hands towards his chest, Dr Jenkins elbowed his way through the swing doors and was gone.

★ ★ ★

*Hell! Now what?* Jake watched as the rest of the surgical team began the painstaking process of closing up his chest. He thought again of Sally. Where was she? Did she know he was here? How would she react? If only he could talk to her—explain that it really wasn't as terrifying as everyone thought... He felt another tug, stronger this time, pulling him back down.

# 15
# Detox deliverance

"I'll start with a short introduction," said Dietrich Detox, standing up and clearing his throat as he looked around the room. All heads turned to him expectantly.

"A directive was issued this morning from Command Central, calling for an immediate detoxification of the entire organism. You all know what happened last week. The organism is in serious trouble and we have to take some drastic measures. As a specialist in toxicology and the chemicals, additives and preservatives in foods, I've been put in charge of this programme." Putting his hands in the pockets of his white lab coat, he paused to let his words sink in.

"This will mean two things. Firstly, all significant parties along the Alimentary Canal are obliged to participate in this programme so that the organism can detoxify."

"What do they mean by 'significant'?" interrupted Pontius Palate.

"Anyone who has anything to do with the processing of food and other substances coming into the organism," said Dietrich. "Any other questions before I continue?" He looked at them challengingly.

There was silence.

"So, as I was saying, this detox programme is mandatory, and will continue for at least 10 weeks—"

"Wait a minute," said Candice Candida. "Why are we being held responsible for all the toxins in the organism? That doesn't seem fair at all. What about all the others? Why just us?"

"You, Sam Stomach, Pontius Palate and all the microorganisms in Colon County," said Dietrich, gesturing at them with an impatient wave of his hand, "play the most significant role in terms of generating certain toxins or a craving for nutritionally empty foods. When you and your various teams proliferate, you create a demand for more sugars and stuff to keep you fed. Then things just get progressively worse for everyone else, impeding the function of almost every department. Look what happened. We almost lost everything."

"I'm just doing my job," said Pontius Palate belligerently. "I don't decide what His Lordship eats. All I do is try to keep the palate clean, keep the Taste Buddies in order, and suffer from the whims of the Eyes & Nose department when they see or hear of something they'd like to sample. What am I being penalized for?"

"You're the reason the rest of us are in trouble, Pontius," said Candice angrily. "You've betrayed us all with your stupid cravings! If it weren't for your sweet palate, and your whole Taste Buddy Team craving sugary things, we wouldn't be in this mess. You've got us all addicted, and now—"

"That's enough!" said Dietrich, exasperated. "Look, no single individual is to blame, here. And you have to understand that something has to be done to prevent a recurrence of what happened this morning. There's such an overload of toxins coming into the system that we simply don't have the manpower to deal with it. It's reaching crisis levels." He paused to remove his jacket. "And you, Pontius," he continued, "create plenty of havoc of your own. You and your Taste Buddies are the first line in the chain of things going wrong. When his Lordship acquires a taste for something, he wants more of it. So it's up to you to nip this in the taste bud, so to speak, and reduce his cravings for sweet, processed stuff. This will give us all a chance to recover."

"Always the fall guy..." muttered Pontius under his breath.

"What's the second thing?" interjected Sam Stomach.

"There will have to be cutbacks and layoffs, depending on how well this initial phase of the programme goes," said Dietrich.

"How do we survive if there are cutbacks?" said Candice, looking stricken.

"That's the whole point," said Dietrich. "You're not all *supposed* to survive. We have to cut back and make sure that every department that's generating toxins is reduced down to a manageable skeleton crew. It's for the survival of the entire organism. Your team, Candice, regularly outnumbers the Friendly Flora that do the cleaning up in here, and we can't afford to have that continue. You all have to detox and downsize, I'm afraid, and there will be no exceptions." He paused for effect, glaring at them all over the rims of his small, round glasses.

"We'll be starting with an outline of the toxin-reduction procedure, before moving on to the cleansing programme—"

"What will that involve, exactly?" said Sam Stomach.

"It will be a 10-week dietary programme designed to reduce consumption of toxic substances, such as sugars, refined starches, deep-fried and processed foods, etc, and to generate a demand for cleaner, more nutritious fuel."

"We're going to starve," moaned Candice.

"And how are we supposed to do this?" asked Sam indignantly. "Just cold turkey?"

"Cold turkey, cold chicken, cold eggs, whatever it takes." said Dietrich. "It won't kill you, Sam. And, if it makes you feel any better, everyone will eventually have to go through this, not just you. Phase II of this programme involves a detox for every department in the organism. So once you've done your part in reducing the demand, they'll be next. Any other questions?"

He was met with glum stares.

"Okay, let's begin. We already have a complete inventory of what comes in and what it contains. So this part of the process is merely to determine where, exactly, the toxic demand is generated so that we can figure out how best it can be curbed." He paused and looked pointedly at Candice, adding, "We're looking for hardened addicts, and there will be no mercy from Command Central for those who refuse to detox and clean up their act." He paused again, consulting his notes. "Pontius, we'll start with your department, since that's where the food first enters the organism. I'll need you to give me a detailed breakdown of everything that passes your palate, and how it is processed in cooperation with the rest of the organism. Go ahead, please," he gestured towards Pontius who was slumped, sulking, in his chair.

"It's not that simple, y'know," said Pontius, chewing on a toothpick. "My job is to identify all the numerous flavours that come in, and then relay that information to the various processing centres below. But certain people make my job very difficult," he glared pointedly at Candice and Sam.

"What's that supposed to mean?" said Candice indignantly, tossing back her blond curls.

"Your little predilection for sweet and starchy things causes a huge backlog of toxins that I have to contend with," said Pontius with disdain. "And I'll have you know that I'm not the one creating these sugar cravings. You and Sam can take the full credit for that one."

"Now, wai—" began Sam.

"Sure, I may have certain preferences when it comes to identifying the various flavours that come in," continued Pontius, undeterred, "but I don't *decide* what comes in. You do. You and your team create such an insatiable appetite for the stuff that you're constantly sending distress signals up to Command, bellyaching for more."

"Pontius, what exactly does this backlog look like?" interjected Dietrich before Sam and Candice could retaliate. "And how do you deal with it?"

"Every morning I wake up to a horrible white coating on everything, and it's just disgusting. There's a rotten smell, too, coming from all that undigested, putrefying stuff that the system just can't handle. It all makes it really hard for me to do my job and correctly identify flavours or possibly injurious foods coming into the system. I try scraping the white stuff off with a broom, but what's needed is a complete change in diet. And the departments further south need to clean up their act."

"Sam, what do you think can be done about this?" asked Dietrich, turning to Sam Stomach.

"Well, firstly, I don't like your tone," said Sam, shaking his finger at Pontius. "I mean, who do you—"

"Sam, let's not take this personally," said Dietrich. "We all need to work together as a team on this if we're to find a solution. Please just give us your input and ideas. I'm sure you've got plenty of good ones."

"Yeah, well, I know what needs to be done," said Sam grudgingly. "Certainly, there needs to be a change in diet, but we also need more manpower to break down the various food groups as they come into the system. We need more enzymes and hydrochloric acid, for starters. Without enough of those, there's a lot of putrefaction going on and that's what causes the build-up of toxins. That causes traffic congestion, and then it's hard for things to get through. Our teams are getting depleted and we need help from the outside."

"Any ideas on how to do that?" said Dietrich, making some notes in his pad.

"I've been sending repeated messages up to Command Centre, but they seem to be having trouble getting the message through to His Lordship. We have to find some other way to reach him... but I haven't figured that out yet." He paused, perplexed. "Until that happens, all we can do is try to reduce our intake and lessen the load we all have to carry."

"Okay, we'll go with that, for now," said Dietrich, scribbling in his pad before turning to Candice. "So, Candice... Candice? Are you all right, Candice?"

Candice was slumped over her notepad, seemingly in a daze.

Sam leaned over and shook her. She grunted in response and slowly lifted her head.

"Whassamatter?" she said, her words slurred. "Is it lunchtime yet?"

"Candice, what's going on?"

"She's having one of her blood-sugar slumps," said Pontius in disgust. "See? I told you. She can't live without the stuff. She's completely hooked."

"I juss need a cookie or shomething," said Candice, her eyelids drooping.

"Okay, let's break for lunch," said Dietrich, exasperated. "We're having chicken salad, with some raw nuts, followed by a protein smoothie this afternoon. The detox diet starts today."

# 16
# Fragile ego-system

"Millie, drop whatever you're doing. I need something right now," said Edgar Ego to his secretary over the intercom. "I want you to find..." he paused to consult his notes, "...Jeremy Gene, and have him sent to my office immediately."

"Yes, Sir," said Millie Me, hastily reaching for her cell phone.

Edgar got up from his large walnut desk, and began pacing the room, his fists clenched. His tall, solid frame seemed to fill the spacious office, despite the full-length mirrors he had had installed along one wall. "I can't believe the incompetence..." he muttered under his breath.

"When I get my hands on that imbecile..." He stopped to examine himself in the glass, stroking his smooth-shaven chin, and running his fingers through his dark, well-groomed hair. He congratulated himself on his new custom-tailored black suit, which looked stunning against his crisp white shirt, and accentuated his deep tan. He beamed at himself appreciatively in the mirror, revealing white, perfectly capped, even teeth. Turning sideways, and sucking in his stomach, he admired his slim profile...

A timid rap at the door interrupted his reverie.

"Yes?" he thundered, the smile gone in a flash. "Come!"

The door opened slowly, and Jeremy peered tremulously into the large room.

"Come IN!" bellowed Edgar, losing all patience, "...and close that door!"

Jeremy sidled around the door, closing it slowly behind him.

"Sit down!" shouted Edgar, gesturing to the chair on the other side of his desk. Jeremy crept along the red carpet, and seated himself gingerly in the black leather chair. On the other side of his desk, Edgar leaned his clenched fists on the polished wood and glared down at Jeremy from his full six feet three inches.

"What do you have to say for yourself?"

"Nothing, Sir, I mean..." Jeremy muttered. "I, eh, can't apologize enough, Sir, for what happened. It's the first time..."

"And definitely your last!" said Edgar, sinking heavily into his polished executive's chair. "Just who do you think you are, playing around with that sensitive equipment, anyway?"

"Well, Lily Liver put me in charge..." began Jeremy.

"Don't you realize what this does to my reputation?" roared Edgar, oblivious to Jeremy's response. "Don't you realize that the entire success of the organism depends on the image that I, personally, maintain?"

"Yes, Sir, I do now," said Jeremy dejectedly, casting his eyes around the room.

"See those pictures there?" shouted Edgar, gesturing to the array of framed photographs lining the plush walls.

Jeremy looked at the numerous shots of Edgar beaming proudly, some with trophies, others showing him being presented with awards by top management, and still others showing him naked from the waist up, revealing his strong, muscular body.

"That's what success looks like, boy," said Edgar. "And you obviously do not have what it takes to get there. You have not only put a serious dent in my overall credibility, but have had the temerity to mess around with my most important asset, which I've spent years building—my masculinity!"

He paused and glared down at Jeremy. "What do you have to say for yourself?"

"I'm a worthless piece of shit, not worthy of your attention, Sir!" said Jeremy, suddenly disgusted and angry at his own timidity. "I'm not even worth your time, Sir, and you should really—"

"DON'T tell me what to do, boy," boomed Edgar. "You're lucky that I haven't had you deported for what you did."

"Yes, Sir," said Jeremy, subdued again. "Maybe, Sir, I could suggest a solution..."

"I doubt it," said Edgar. "But let's hear it anyway."

"Perhaps I could help out voluntarily with this new Toxins Anonymous programme, helping Dietrich get the whole organism cleaned up…"

"That's far too easy a solution," said Edgar, narrowing his eyes, and making Jeremy squirm in his seat. "I have something else in mind for you." He reached for his briefcase, withdrawing a slim file. "Take this and study it," he said, shoving it in Jeremy's direction. "There's a map in there, and instructions on where to go, but after that you're on your own."

"Well, can you tell me just a little about what I'm supposed to do?" asked Jeremy, a sense of foreboding creeping up his spine.

"There's an inexplicable phenomenon occurring in the Solar Plexus Centre that we need to have checked out. No one knows what's involved, so we're assuming it's a high-risk operation, and one that can only be handled by someone as imminently expendable as you." Edgar smiled at him coldly.

"But what happens if I can't handle it?" asked Jeremy, anxiety twisting his insides. "I mean, is there no one who can help me with this?"

"No," said Edgar. "That's the whole point. This is your one chance to redeem yourself, so you'd better make it good. Now get out of my sight before I change my mind and think of something worse." With that, he turned to his phone and began to dial, ignoring Jeremy as he quietly left the office.

Head hanging forlornly, file in hand, Jeremy closed the door softly behind him. As he walked slowly down the corridor, he heard Edgar's booming voice call after him: "And report back to me when you've finished, boy!"

# 17
# Soul searching

By the time Jeremy reached Lily Liver's department, he had worked himself into a rage and was ready to do some serious damage. Map in hand, he stormed into her office. "It's easy to see where you got your name," he yelled at her. "You put me doing a job I couldn't possibly do right, and then went off and left me to face the music. I call that downright cowardly and lily-livered. And now—"

"Jeremy, sit down, and let's talk about this," Lily said quietly, taking off her glasses and leaning back in her swivel chair. "You didn't just have problems with Edgar, you were also dealing with your own overblown ego and we can't have that, in here. You can't go strutting around pontificating about spiritual values when you don't practise them yourself. Being a spiritual being requires humility, which seems to be in short supply right now." She sat silently as he digested this.

"But what you did was wrong, surely," said Jeremy, annoyed at having the tables so quickly turned on him. "I didn't deserve that kind of humiliation."

"Often, that's the only thing that can break through huge pride and force us to see what's really going on."

"Well, that didn't seem to work with Edgar," said Jeremy petulantly. "How come he wasn't brought to his knees since he's the one so filled with ego?"

"It's his job to flaunt his ego," said Lily, patiently. "Ego is designed for the survival of the organism, and without it we would all be dead. Ego is largely fear, but in terms of personal safety and security, it's what keeps the organism from endangering itself. The ego has to be strong enough to be the overriding instinct in times of threat or danger. And it's our job to work with that and make sure that we obey all those survival instincts that the ego generates. It also serves to make the organism the best it can be—physically, mentally and in other ways—which helps us all to fulfill our greater potential. So, now, what else were you going to tell me?"

Pursing his lips, Jeremy looked at her defiantly for a moment, then unfolded his map on the desk.

"He gave me this and told me to find out what's going on in the Solar Plexus area. But I haven't a clue what to do once I get there."

"Go there with humility and honest questions and you can't go wrong. Now, let me get back to work. We're swamped with this detox programme and I'm short-staffed as it is... Unless you want to help me out again, in some other department...?"

"No way," said Jeremy, hurriedly, getting out of his chair. "But..."

"That's all you need, Jeremy—humility," said Lily with a dismissive wave of her hand. "Now go and take care of your assignment and see if you can gain some enlightenment along the way."

"One more thing," says Jeremy, pausing at the doorway. "Who's normally in charge of the Penis Panel? I mean, who should have been doing the night shift that got me into this mess?"

"Percy P, but he badly needed a holiday. Edgar would only allow it if I managed to get someone else to stand in while Percy got some rest. Any other questions?" Not waiting for an answer, Lily returned her attention to the files on her desk.

"I can't take much more of this brow beating," Jeremy muttered to himself as he left the Liver Department. He stopped to glance at his map again, and plotted his route to Solar Plexus Centre. It looked as if it was about 150 cells southeast of where he was right now, so it should only take him about half an hour to get there. Folding up the map again and stuffing his hands into his trouser pockets, he set off. He had only gone about five blocks, when he saw an eerie yellow light glowing in the distance. He stopped, looked around, but there was no one in sight. He'd just have to keep going alone. As he walked, the light grew stronger, and he felt a strange tingling sensation prickling his spine. His hair seemed to be standing on end and he could swear that someone was actually touching his head, and moving his hair from side to side. He ran his fingers hurriedly through his hair, thinking of spiders or other creepy crawlies, but there was nothing, and the tingling got steadily stronger.

He passed a sign for Solar Plexus Central—another 20 cells to the right, it said. Taking a deep breath, he rounded the corner and was suddenly enveloped in a blazing light so dazzling that it obliterated all other landmarks. All he could see was thick yellow light, and now he could feel that tingling sensation all over his body. His hair stood on end, his stomach churned, he wanted to turn and run, but his feet seemed rooted to the ground. He didn't know what this 'thing' was, but it was powerful and he didn't like it. How could he possibly fight something like this? It didn't even have a form. It was just one huge big energy field. He should just start walking slowly backwards and—

"Jeremy." He jumped as the voice echoed all around him. He couldn't tell where it was coming from; it was as if it was coming from the light itself, but that was impossible...

"Jeremy, can you hear me?"

"Uh, yes, I can hear you, whoever you are. Who ARE you?" Jeremy scanned the light on all sides, but could see nothing through the yellow fog.

"I am the soul," said the voice. "I am the higher aspect of this organism and I am here to teach you."

"About hu... humility?" asked Jeremy, trying to flatten his electrified hair.

"Among other things," replied the voice. "The organism is in trouble and I have been called in to help."

"But what has that got to do with me?" said Jeremy. "How can I do anything? I'm a nothing in this place. I've just been sent here as the fall guy, the expendable one."

"Not so, Jeremy. I need to get some messages through to the rest of the organism so as to restore balance in the system, and you will play an important role in that. Without divine intervention, the organism strays too much into the mental and physical regions and neglects the signs and messages that I am trying to transmit at more subtle levels—signs that eventually take the form of ill-health and physical symptoms if not heeded in time."

"I've heard about you," said Jeremy, filled with a sense of awe and wonder. "But I didn't think anyone ever got to actually *meet* you. I mean, aren't you supposed to be invisible and live in heaven, or something?"

"Well, in a way, I *am* heaven," replied the soul. "But I am also a part of you. When you are in tune with me, you are fulfilling your purpose here on earth and you are happy, healthy, joyful, creative, prosperous, loving, beloved beings, connected to source and other living things, and at peace with your world. What could be more heavenly than that?"

"Not much, I suppose." Jeremy considered for a moment. "But does that mean that you have to meditate for hours every day and give up things like chocolate cake and... and... well, girlfriends, and watching violent action movies and stuff like that?"

"It's not quite that simple. Meditating alone would not be enough to cleanse your mind. And eliminating things like chocolate cake from your diet would not be enough to purify your body. The organism is infinitely more complex than that. Sit down for a moment and I'll give you an idea of what I'm talking about."

Jeremy sat, crossing his legs.

"Now close your eyes and take a few deep breaths. Let your body relax, and feel yourself connected to the ground. Think of one of those violent movies you mentioned, and see what you feel."

Jeremy concentrated, remembering the latest action film he had seen. All of a sudden, the yellow energy around him seemed to diminish and turn cold. He shivered.

"What happened?"

"You diminished your own life force," replied the soul. "You were focussing on something negative and life-threatening, even if it was only fiction, and that lessened the expression of your soul, which is ultimately the highest expression of love. Now, this time think of something you love. It could be someone in your family, a girlfriend, or even an animal you kept as a pet. Focus on that and see what you feel."

Again Jeremy concentrated, focussing this time on his grandmother and the feelings he had experienced when he was with her as a child. Immediately, the tingling sensation increased and he could feel a warm glow from the swirling yellow energy around him. He felt warm, strong, protected and content. And, for some reason, he felt hot tears prickling behind his closed eyelids.

"What was *that*?" he said, fighting back the tears.

"That was merely the expression of your love," said the soul gently. "Let yourself feel your grandmother's love, and the love you had for her. Don't fight it."

"How did you know I was thinking about her?" Jeremy felt his cheeks grow hot, as if he had been caught doing something bad.

"We are one, Jeremy. And there is no shame in feeling your emotions. That is what makes you human." There was silence for a moment before the voice continued.

"Do you see how that feeling differs from the negative thoughts that you were focussing on earlier? Do you see how it nourishes and uplifts you, making you feel good inside? It connects you with others and with your higher self. And it also helps you to let go of old hurts, to feel your emotions, and to have compassion for others who may have hurt you in the past. Being in that state most of the time is the ultimate goal of all beings."

"Yes, but if that's all there is to it, why doesn't everyone do this? All I did was think of someone I loved..."

"Humans have a very short memory, and they become very attached to material things that distract them from these other divine aspects of themselves. They are so filled with fear of not being accepted and of not being able to survive in this world that they forget all about their true essence. They are spiritual beings trying to have a physical experience, yet most live their lives as if they were physical beings doing their utmost to avoid any kind of spiritual experience."

"But why would they do that, when it doesn't make them happy?"

"Spirit is power," said the soul. "That is where our power comes from. Yet if we embraced our power, we would have to become the beings we were born to be, and that can be scary."

"Why? Why is that scary?" asked Jeremy. "Doesn't everyone want to be powerful? Don't they want to be all they can be?"

"Some do, but most are conditioned by their upbringing to stay small and insignificant in the world and they find it very difficult to believe that they could be powerful. So they learn not to shine too brightly if they want to stay out of trouble. Society has created the belief that there is safety in numbers. If we all believe the same thing, we are told, and act the same way, then we'll be safe and there will be harmony and happiness. But this supposed safety costs us our individual freedom of expression and individuality. We die inside when we have to conform and cannot express our uniqueness."

"What about me? I don't know what I'm supposed to be doing, or who I am, or anything. I don't even know what I want, so how do I figure out what to do with my life?"

"You keep doing what you just did—connecting with your heart and feeling what's in there. With practice, you will dig beneath the layers of fear and self-doubt to discover what's underneath. And with faith—in yourself, in your soul and in God, which are really all the same thing—you will get there. But you must want it. It is not a journey to be undertaken lightly because you will face opposition and will be challenged in your conviction once you start to be your true self."

"But why? Why should anyone care if I'm myself? They can live their own life and I won't bother them."

"When you start to discover who you are, you force those around you to change also. If you are no longer behaving as you were 'supposed' to, then they can no longer relate to you in the same way. This causes change to occur and it can be very unsettling for those who do not want to change and grow. But it is the ultimate gift. Being yourself is what you are here to be. What else is there?"

Jeremy reflected. "Well, food brings us a lot of pleasure, and then there's nature, and... and sex, I suppose," he said, blushing.

"But they are all part of divine creation, not separate from it. They are a means of expressing your divine self. In fact, those are things that are expressly designed to bring you closer to God and your soul. Without them there would be no wonder, no appreciation for beauty, no love for your body, and no pleasure in joining with another human being at the highest possible level. It is how these things are used that matters, and it is through our wise use of them that we have the opportunity to reach greater heights of fulfillment and bliss."

"I always knew there was something rather spiritual about chocolate cake," said Jeremy, laughing nervously. He was feeling a little uncomfortable with all this talk of bliss.

"But you just eat your cake and then it's gone. There is nothing terribly spiritual about that," said the soul.

"What do you mean? Isn't that what you're supposed to do with chocolate cake? I thought you just said food was spiritual." Jeremy was starting to get a bit impatient. This conversation was going round in circles and he was supposed to figure out why this soul thing was here and then report back to Edgar. If he didn't get back soon—

"Jeremy. Think for a moment about that slice of chocolate cake. Think about all the things that have to happen just for it to be created. Think of the sunshine and good soil that are required to grow the wheat, cocoa and other ingredients, of the farmers who have to tend the crops in the fields, of the cows that are raised for the milk, and of the truck drivers who have to transport those goods across the country. Think about the bakers who get up at 5am to bake these delicious things for you and think of the sales people who stand behind the counter and sell these cakes all day long. Think about what the body has to do to process this rich food—of the stomach that has to coat it in acids and enzymes from the liver and pancreas so that it can be broken down and converted into energy to run your body—and of all the millions of cellular activities that have to take place to process the by-products of this one slice of cake. Think of all—"

"Whoa! Okay, okay, I get the message." Jeremy shifted uncomfortably on the ground, feeling a wave of guilt wash over him.

"So how do you feel about chocolate cake, now?" asked the voice. "Do you think you'll wolf it down without another thought the next time you take a bite?"

"I feel rather humble and ashamed, actually," said Jeremy quietly. "And chocolate cake will never be the same again."

"Good. Then that's enough for today."

"Wait! Don't go. I've been sent here on a mission, and I have to know what to do next. What about Edgar Ego, and what about the survival of the organism and—?"

"Just go back and tell them all in your own words what we talked about today and you should see some changes." The yellow light began to ebb, and Jeremy could feel the energy diminish.

"No, wait, please. I'll be in terrible trouble if I don't go back with more than that. What do I tell Edgar? He'll be furious that I just spent all this time talking about chocolate cake and action movies and my Granny. He'll have me kicked out, he'll—"

"Jeremy, don't let your fear overwhelm your love. You are part of me and I am part of you. We co-create together, so you can bring about changes, too, just by changing yourself. Think on that as you walk home, and I'm sure you'll find the answers to your questions. We'll talk again soon."

"Just one more thing! What do I...?" But the swirling yellow energy had vanished almost as suddenly as it had appeared, and Jeremy was left standing alone, his own voice echoing back to him in the empty darkness.

# 18
# Back from the brink

"I had a *coronary* for God's sake—a bypass at 35! My life is ruined!" said Jake, staring at the white ceiling in his hospital room. "Not to mention my career and my health."

"You're alive, Jake, and that's all that matters right now," said Sally, biting back the tears that threatened to overwhelm her again. "Plenty of people your age go on to live long and healthy lives, provided they take care of themselves. It's just a wake-up call. That's all. You must be positive and just focus on getting strong and healthy so that this doesn't happen again. It's a wonderful gift, really."

"Oh, please, Sal. Spare me the New Age philosophy..." Jake looked off into space.

"Fine," said Sally curtly, getting up and reaching for her coat.

"I'm sorry, Sal. I didn't mean that. Please don't go. How did you know I was in here, anyway?"

"Charlie called me. Someone from the office called him as soon as they heard."

"Oh. Right. I'm glad you're here, Sal. Look, I'm sorry about what happened the other night. I was stressed and needed some time to think. We can talk about that when I'm out of here. Right now, I need to figure out what's going on. I don't even know what caused this. I feel completely ignorant and powerless. And now I don't know if I can ever trust my heart again..."

He looked at her. "...or your love for me."

Sally adjusted her coat on her arm as if gauging her commitment.

"Please, Sal, can you try to explain what caused this? I want to get back in control of my health."

Sally sat back down on the chair, folding her coat across her knees and studying its big brown buttons.

"Sal, I'm asking for your help, here, and I'm open to input, okay? "

Sally sighed and took a deep breath. "Well, there are lots of different schools of thought on this. But, from what I've seen, it often starts with some kind of inflammation in the arteries, which can be caused by infection, bad food or stress—all of which cause a depletion of certain essential nutrients. And when the arteries get inflamed, the liver produces more cholesterol to patch up the inflamed spots, and then those patches get calcified so that they don't slip off. If this didn't happen, the blood vessels could burst from the inflammation. So cholesterol is not all bad, although most people don't realize this."

"But what about all that cholesterol building up? Surely that's the cause of the problem, blocking the arteries and causing the coronary, right?" Frustrated, Jake ran his hands through his hair.

"Well, yes," Sally admitted. "But the real problem is the reason for the inflammation in the first place. The blood vessels get inflamed when there are not enough natural anti-inflammatories in the body to prevent inflammation."

"So what are these anti-inflammatories?"

"They're called omega-3s, and you can get them from certain foods such as fish oils."

"So I just have to eat more of those and I'll be fine? Sounds awfully simple, Sal."

Jake folded his arms across his chest, and frowned at her skeptically.

"It's not that simple," said Sally. "You have to do other things, too, such as eating right in general, cleansing your liver and getting enough protein so that your immune system is strong and you don't get infections or too much degeneration in the system—"

"I've been on the other side," Jake said quietly, examining the folds on the white bedspread.

"What… what do you mean, 'on the other side'?" Sally sat back abruptly in her chair.

"I left my body and was looking down on myself from above," said Jake softly, turning to face her. "I saw them operating on me. It was okay, Sal. I felt no pain. My only concern was for you. I couldn't leave you down here alone. So I came back. You brought me back."

"Didn't you want to ...to come back?" Sally's chest was heaving. "Are you s...s...sorry you did?"

"No, darling, of course not," said Jake, raising his head off the pillow and clasping her hand tightly. "I mean, of course I'm not sorry. I will go back there eventually, I suppose, no matter how healthy I get." He smiled at her. "But it's obviously not my time yet. I've still got things to do here—with you. And it was wonderful to know that dying is really not that bad. I won't ever be afraid of it again."

Sally stared at him, her throat working as she digested this.

"It's funny, you know," Jake continued. "Not being afraid of death somehow makes living an awful lot nicer. And a hell of a lot more meaningful."

He relaxed back onto the pillow and regarded her fondly.

"It's good to be back." As he said it, he realized that it was true. "I've been given a second chance. And I know there's more to life than this..." He gestured to the plain hospital room around them. "I want to live differently. I want to start from scratch again and get it right, this time."

# 19
# Toxic treatment

Scores of bottles lined the shelves. Some contained strange-colored liquids, and others held powders. All were labeled with numbers. To one side, a laboratory technician was leaning over a Bunsen burner, stirring a steaming, murky-looking liquid in a glass dish. In the middle of the room stood Dietrich in his white coat, facing the group seated before him. "Silence, please," he said, rapping his ruler against the long conference table. "Today we are going to start Part II of the detox programme. We'll be learning about additives and preservatives in foods, as well as environmental toxins such as heavy metals and pesticides." He gestured to the bottles behind him. "These are the various chemicals, additives, preservatives and other toxins we'll be looking at, and this..." he gestured to his technician on his right, "...is Terry from Toxicology. He will be showing you some of the chemical reactions that take place within the organism when these various substances are ingested. Now, let's begin."

"What's the point?" said Oliver abruptly. "I mean, why should we bother learning about all this stuff if his Lordship is totally unaware of it and just keeps eating hamburgers and smoking cigarettes?"

"Ideally, we do want to make him aware of these issues and try to get him to change his eating habits and lifestyle," said Dietrich. "And that's a major project that's in the works, apparently. But, in the meantime, unless we know how to process these substances, we will soon be overwhelmed with the backlog and unable to cope. Each department needs to know exactly what to do when one of these substances comes in, and then we must all coordinate with Command Central to ensure that we work effectively as a team."

He looked around the table. "Any other questions?" He paused for a split second before continuing. "Okay. So, let's begin by looking at the main departments responsible for this area of detoxification. There's you, Oliver, together with Lily and the rest of her staff, in the Liver Department, which is responsible for almost 500 functions. Many of these are to do with cleansing, as we'll see. Oliver, why don't you fill us in on some of the details."

"No problem," said Oliver, standing up and looking around the room. "Our department is actually the largest organ in the entire organism and is the only one that can regenerate itself when a part of it gets damaged. We're pretty proud of that, actually. Even if a quarter of our department is removed, it will grow back to its original shape and size in a short time. Quite amazing, isn't it?"

"Oliver, just stick to the facts, please," said Dietrich impatiently. "We're not here to glorify your existence."

"Sorry," said Oliver, clearing his throat. "Well, we have many functions, as Dietrich pointed out, one of the most important of which is probably the secretion of bile, which is necessary for the digestion of fats. Bile is stored in the gallbladder department, and it breaks fat down into small globules. It is also needed for the absorption of fat-soluble vitamins A, D, E, F and K, and helps to assimilate calcium—"

"Oliver," Dietrich interrupted again, exasperated. "This is a detox programme, not a biology class. Please just get to the point."

"Right. Sorry, Dietrich. Just got a bit carried away there. Well, the liver acts as a detoxifier. When protein metabolism and bacterial fermentation of food in the intestines produce the by-product ammonia, we detoxify it. But we also combine toxic substances, such as metabolic waste, insecticide residues, drugs, alcohol and chemicals, with other substances that are less toxic. Together, these are excreted through the kidneys. So, you see, we're indispensable to the entire organism..." Catching sight of Dietrich's expression, he stopped and hastily sat down.

"That's about it, Dietrich, I think."

"Thank you, Oliver," said Dietrich, turning back to the rest of the group. "Billy, maybe you'd like to elaborate a bit on your department."

"Yes, Dietrich, no problem." Billy Gallbladder stood up slowly, a short, stocky figure with a quiet, self-assured face. "Our department, like many others here, is fundamental to the well-being of the organism. We store bile, a powerful fat-emulsifying substance that the liver department makes from cholesterol. When things are going well, we work with flawless precision, releasing bile (as Oliver mentioned), just when it's needed to help digest food. We also absorb nutrients and keep cholesterol levels in check. Although many people think that eating fat and cholesterol leads to gallstones, in fact, eating too little fat—the good kind—and too many carbohydrates in the form of grains, sugars and starches, actually leads to trouble in our department."

He looked at his notes.

"We have one fundamental purpose, on the physical level: to help digest food, especially fats. If we don't get enough fat to keep us in good working order, we just get stuck with all that bile sitting there losing water and thickening. Not very nice stuff."

He looked at his colleagues, an expression of benign reproach on his calm face.

"On the emotional level, probably our most important function is our influence on decision-making. And I'll explain that more in a moment. We also have an important effect on dreams."

He looked at Dietrich.

"I'd like to try to put things in perspective so that you can all get a better idea of the big picture, and see how we can best interact during this programme. If you'll bear with me a moment, Dietrich…"

Dietrich nodded for him to continue.

"We've all been looking at the purely physical aspect of our work here, but of course there's much more to all of us than that. Every department also has an emotional aspect, which is equally important. We only have to look at how we are affected by what others say or think to realize that the whole system can become upset and inefficient if it is emotionally challenged."

He looked around the table, pausing a little longer, it seemed, when he came to Sam and Oliver.

"Here's how it works. As Lily knows, her department is, not surprisingly, given its multitude of functions, responsible for the ability to plan life. So it plays quite a significant role in how things operate and how the big picture unfolds. Heather's department, on the other hand, oversees all mental functions, as well as emotional ones. Now, I know that may come as a bit of a surprise to some of you, but think for a moment of how both the mind and the heart usually work together when making any kind of decision."

He paused again, letting the others digest this.

"The upper sections of Highway 22 bring clarity and wisdom to the decision-making process, distinguishing between what's toxic and what's healthy, so everyone in that department works closely with Lily. And my department provides the courage and capacity to make those decisions. All of these functions must be in balance for things to work smoothly. If my department is weak, we all suffer from timidity, and a lack of courage and initiative. I'm responsible for providing the drive and passion to excel and the potential for taking the action required to bring things to fruition. Dealing with adversity is also part of my department's brief. By staying strong, we can be of particular help to you, Heather, among others."

He turned to Dietrich.

"I hope that's helpful, Dietrich."

"Yes, thank you, Billy. I think we can all see the importance of working as a team and not allowing ourselves to get upset."

He looked pointedly at those around the table.

"I have a question for Billy, Dietrich," said Heather.

Dietrich gestured for her to go ahead.

"What about your effect on dreams, Billy? I'm curious to know how that works."

"Ah, yes, Heather. Thanks for reminding me. Our department

has a significant effect on the quality and length of sleep. If we are below par, then the organism will tend to wake up very early and not be able to get back to sleep. And when we are not operating optimally, the organism will tend to have dreams about conflicts, trials and suicide. It's fairly widely known that certain foods and emotions have an effect on dreams, but few people realize that our department does, too. In both cases, of course, there is an imbalance that needs to be addressed."

"Thank you, Billy." Dietrich scanned the room again.

"Now who's next? Karl and Kyla. Which one of you would like to explain about the Kidney Department?"

"She will..." began Karl.

"He will..." said Kyla simultaneously.

"Okay," said Karl, laughing. "I'll do it." He cleared his throat. "As glandular organs, we are primarily responsible for separating waste products from the blood and excreting them as urine. Although some wastes are processed by the liver, as Oliver said, and then go into the intestines via the bile duct."

"But we need lots of pure water to do our job properly," Kyla interjected, "especially when the body needs to detox."

"Yes," said Karl. "That's the biggest problem, Dietrich, and I'm glad we finally have a chance to talk about this. The whole organism is chronically dehydrated and that makes our job very difficult. In fact, there's not much point in doing any of this—" Karl sweeps his arm around the room to indicate all the departments present, "if we can't fix this problem first."

"How can we best address this, Karl?" said Dietrich.

"Well, the first thing is to create thirst, which normally happens automatically when there's not enough water coming in. But the problem is that His Lordship has been ignoring the signal for so long that he no longer knows he's thirsty. And that's when things get dicey." He pauses, looking around the table.

"Go on, please, Karl," prompts Dietrich. "What happens then?"

"Well, if it goes on long enough—and, believe me, it has— the cells begin to shrivel and malfunction and tissues begin to dry out. Brain cells are the most susceptible to dehydration, so confusion and even coma can occur. But Kyla and I feel it too because we play such a key role in processing fluids. His Lordship needs to be drinking at least two litres of water a day to keep things healthy and prevent kidney stones."

"How much would you say we're getting, Karl?"

"Nowhere near that. More like half a litre, if we're lucky, and half of that's either coffee or some kind of sugary drink that only creates more work. Two-thirds of the system is made up of water, you know. But it's not just about keeping the system clean, Dietrich. We lose important mineral salts such as sodium, potassium and chloride, and then water can't move easily from inside the cells into the blood. And that means that the amount of water circulating in the bloodstream gets reduced and blood pressure can drop. This makes His Lordship light-headed, particularly if he stands up suddenly—but he just thinks he needs to eat. He needs to drink! And I don't mean beer. Why can't he understand that? I mean, is there anything simpler than drinking a glass of water every few hours?" Karl pauses for breath, taking out his hanky and mopping his face. "Thing is, Dietrich, if this continues, blood pressure can fall dangerously low, seriously damaging our equipment as well as Lily's and Brian's. So we need to somehow get His Lordship to start tanking up on the H20 so we can get things working the way they should."

"Okay, thank you, Karl. Let me talk to Brian about that and maybe we can come up with a strategy for getting His Lordship to drink more. Suggestions welcome, everyone." Dietrich glances around the table and makes a note in his pad. "Anything to add to that, Kyla?"

"Well, um, yes. We need to make sure that protein gets properly broken down so that things don't clog up the system. Karl and I are often accused of not doing a good job, but we can only be effective if things come to us in the right form. If protein molecules are too large, we can't process them through the system, and this can cause a serious problem."

"Suggestions?" says Dietrich.

"Yes. Better breakdown of protein higher up the system would be the answer, Dietrich—which means more digestive enzymes, as Sam pointed out at our last meeting, so I guess that's being handled."

"Good. Thank you, Kyla and Karl," said Dietrich. "What about you, Sophie? We haven't heard from you in a while."

All eyes turned to Sophie Spleen, sitting quietly at one end of the table.

"Well," said Sophie hesitantly, getting to her feet, "I'll do my best. My partner Mandy Bone Marrow is in Command Central today, venting about the backlog, but she should be joining us later on." She shuffled some papers in front of her on the desk. "Our unit is part of the lymphatic department, and we're based in the upper left part of the abdomen. We're responsible for modifying the blood structure and fighting infection. We help filter out waste products from the body, but we need cooperation from the outside—in the form of movement and exercise—to help us move impurities into the blood for elimination. When there is not enough movement, waste can build up in the unit, causing disease."

She paused, looking around the table before continuing.

"We have another important dimension, related to an individual's self-confidence and self-esteem. So, when the organ is weak, self-confidence may be lacking: likewise, when self-confidence or self-esteem is diminished, our department may be weakened in its natural function. And, as Mandy demonstrates all too often, we spend a lot of time venting so that things don't build up to crisis point."

She looked at Dietrich. "That's it," she said softly, sitting back down in her chair.

"Thank you, Sophie. Well, I think we've done enough for now. Here's what I want you to do for next week."

He looked around the table.

"Sam, I want you to try reducing the appetite levels so that less food comes into the system, and work on boosting hydrochloric levels with Burnie and his team. Oliver, I'd like you and Lily to clean out your unit as much as possible, working with the enzyme squad to ensure clear pathways for enzyme delivery and sufficient amounts of all the various enzymes needed to fully break down whatever comes into the system. Candice, I want you to go on a sugar-free diet and cut out all those sweet pastries and chocolates you eat. Pontius, while we work on reducing the toxic load, I'd like you to try to clear the backlog of bacteria and putrefaction in your unit, and try to encourage the Taste Buddies to acquire a taste for healthier, more savoury foods. Kyla and Karl, could you please inform Command Central that you need lots more pure water coming in and see if they can amp up the thirst factor for this. And Sophie, I'd like you and Mandy to also speak to Command to see if you can programme the organism to get more exercise."

He surveyed the table again, challenging them to complain. 'And I want you all to please consider what else you can do in your respective units to minimize the damage caused to the organism, and to facilitate this detoxification over the next few months."

"But doesn't that depend on His Lordship?" asked Oliver. "I mean, without his cooperation, we can do nothing."

"Yes, Oliver, that's the whole point," said Dietrich. "I need you to stimulate change, to bring about a desire for change on the outside by generating certain needs and impulses on the inside. Hopefully, then, His Lordship will get the message and realize what he must do."

He gathered up his papers amid groans of protest, and put his glasses in his front pocket.

"Good luck, team. I'll see you back here at the same time next week."

# 20
## Side-stepping love

"So. What should I be eating and what should I avoid?" Jake looked at her over the rim of his glass of mineral water.

"Figure it out," said Sally, curtly. She was watering her plants in the living room, going from one to the other, avoiding his gaze.

"What?" Jake looked at her, shocked. "What do you mean? Hey, I thought you wanted me to get healthy and strong."

"That would be nice," said Sally, bending down to water a large rubber plant. "But you can figure it out yourself. You were the one who told me I shouldn't interfere, remember?"

"But..." Perplexed, Jake put down his glass and walked over to her. "What is it, Sal? What's wrong? This isn't like you. Have I done something wrong?"

"Apart from almost dying, you mean?" Sally shot back, anger glinting in her eyes.

"I didn't exactly do it on purpose, you know," Jake said gently, taking the watering can from her and setting it down on the carpet.

"Yes, you did! You did everything you possibly could to completely overload your system. It was guaranteed to explode, at some point. You couldn't have done it better if you'd tried."

"Sal, come and sit down over here so we can talk about this. We were going to talk anyway, before I went into hospital."

He took her arm, but she shrugged him off angrily.

"It's the perfect set-up, isn't it?"

"That's crazy, Sal. For heaven's sake—"

"You're right! It IS crazy. And I'm sick of it!" said Sally, her anger flaring. "It's always the same with men. What makes them think they can just eat what they like, drink gallons of beer, have a potbelly, get horribly unfit, and still be attractive to women, let alone healthy? I mean, the sheer physics of it all is ludicrous, not to mention the arrogance—"

"Hang on a sec—" Jake began.

"It's such a double standard," Sally started pacing around the room. "Women are supposed to keep themselves beautiful for men, yet men go to no such trouble for women because women are conditioned to accept so much less from the opposite sex. And men have no such standards to aspire towards. You don't see men plastered all over billboards or draped over flashy cars looking sexy to entice women. It's all about women enticing men, and being gorgeous enough and slim enough or young and nubile enough to meet their needs. When have you ever heard a man say, *'Oh my God, what woman will have me now! I've put on two inches on my waistline and I've got a double chin'*? Some woman will want them, even if they end up paying in some subtle way. Some woman will be needy enough, and with low enough self-esteem to settle for that and consider herself lucky."

Jake was silent, watching her as she continued to pace.

"Men are so blinkered," Sally continued, her face flushed. "They think that all their sex appeal hangs below the belt, and they don't give any thought to what's above it. They think that if they can perform in bed, the rest won't matter. Their essential manliness will compensate for their indulgences, and for the 'love handles' that result. It's disgusting and it's demeaning to women."

Spent, she flopped down on the couch, arms folded across her chest.

"Is that what happened to you, Sal? Do you feel cheated by me?"

Sally was silent, her eyes exploring the velour of the couch.

"You do, don't you, Sal. That's what this is all about, isn't it?"

"What difference does it make?" Sally said flatly. "You've had a scare, you'll be careful for a while, and then you'll go back to the way you were, eating badly, drinking, not getting enough exercise, putting work first as a good legitimate excuse for not taking care of your body, and thinking you're doing your part as a man because you're earning money, you have a woman, and you can still perform in bed ...most days."

"Ouch," said Jake.

The wooden clock on the wall measured the silence between them.

"And what if I truly *do* want to change, Sal?" said Jake, sitting down beside her. "What then?"

Holding her close, he stroked her hair, and kissed her cheek. She felt wooden in his arms, and he hugged her tighter, murmuring in her ear.

"You know what, Sal? I think everything you said is true. There are double standards. I see that now. Almost dying has shown me just how complacent and arrogant I've been, thinking I was invincible. I see that I wasn't taking responsibility for myself and that created a kind of power vacuum that you got sucked into. It wasn't fair. I should have had stronger, healthier boundaries." He paused, took her chin in his hands and turned her face towards him. "I love you, Sal. You're what I came back for. I want to build a life with you. I want to have a life of meaning and fulfillment. I want passion and love. I don't want to go back to being the way I was."

"Fine," Sally said, turning away from him, her voice tight. "Whatever."

"I'm so sorry for the pain I caused you. I was an idiot. I had no regard for my body, my health, my self, my life with you, my true calling. I deserved to die."

An anguished wail burst forth from Sally, making him jump. Heart pounding, he held her to his chest, rocking her to and fro, waiting.

"I hate you!" she told his sweater. "I thought you were dead. I don't want to be responsible for you any more. You can fix yourself. I don't care."

"Yes, you do, darling. You care lots," said Jake softly. "You were never responsible for me, but you tried to do the job I should have been doing for myself. And you only hate me because you love me."

"Rubbish," said Sally, her voice muffled by the sweater. Abruptly she sat up and looked at him. "I will never love you again," she swore passionately, her eyes flashing. "I will never, ever have anything to do with a man who is not fit, healthy, responsible—"

"...perfect, you mean?" asked Jake gently.

"Yes, bloody perfect!" said Sally. She looked at him, her mouth quivering.

"You love me, Sal. I can feel it," said Jake, placing his hand gently on her heart.

"Well, I don't want to," wailed Sally, collapsing into his arms. "I'll unlove you. I would have had to anyway, if you had died."

"You can't unlove me," said Jake. "And if you try to, I'll just love you all the more. And I'll get so sickeningly healthy that you'll be stuck with me for eternity. Then what?"

Sally looked at him, her lower lip quivering again.

Jake pulled her to him and kissed her till all the barriers were gone.

# 21
# Truth and inspiration

A sea of faces swam before him and his knees felt like jelly. Jeremy had no idea what he was going to say, or how he was even going to remain upright long enough to say it. Surveying the vast auditorium before him, he saw that people were still milling in, looking for empty seats and chattering noisily among themselves. He felt sick to his stomach, and there was no way that—

"Over here, boy!" Edgar yelled at him, gesturing impatiently towards the podium in the middle of the stage. "Stand on this and make sure you speak clearly." Edgar pointed towards the small platform behind the podium, and Jeremy approached it slowly, his feet leaden and his expression one of miserable defeat. As he climbed up onto the platform, Edgar raised his hand towards the crowd and the chattering gradually died down. Jeremy was gazing out at an audience of over 300, most of whom he didn't know, and almost all of whom were in more senior positions than he was. They looked expectant and serious.

"Ladies and gentlemen," Edgar began. "We have asked you here this evening for what promises to be a fascinating dissertation on the strange phenomenon that has been observed in the Solar Plexus Centre recently. I sent Jeremy Gene here..." he gestured magnanimously towards the podium, "...on a mission to investigate this phenomenon, and this evening he will give you his personal account of what he discovered." He turned back towards Jeremy again, giving an imperious nod as he resumed his seat at the back of the stage.

There was a hush in the auditorium. The only thing Jeremy could hear was his heart pounding in his chest, and his ears ringing from the pressure. *So this is what terror feels like*, he thought. He rubbed his sweaty palms on his trousers and shot a desperate glance at Lily, who he could see sitting in the front row. She smiled, nodding her encouragement, and waited. They all waited. He could hear Edgar clearing his throat behind him, a subtle hint to get on with it, and he fought to control his panic. Taking a deep breath, he found himself praying—something he hadn't done for a very long time. Please God, tell me what to say. I need help. I can't do this. Please...

Suddenly, his scalp began to tingle and he felt himself surrounded by the same electricity he had experienced when he went to meet the soul. It gave him goose bumps and made his hair stand on end. But he felt comforted. *I'm here*, said a voice in his head. *You're not alone. Just speak from the heart and you'll be fine.*

Jeremy looked around, half expecting to see the bright light beside him, but there was nothing—just empty space filled with the tangible sense of expectancy from the crowd before him.

"Em, I'd like to tell you about my meeting with the soul," he began, his voice cracking. Clearing his throat and taking a sip of water from the beaker on the podium, he continued hesitantly. "I didn't really believe that the soul existed as something tangible, although I'd heard and read a lot about it. I thought it was just a concept—something to give us a sense of security or hope, maybe. But I never thought I could actually *meet* one, let along have a conversation with it."

There was a general murmur from the crowd, but Jeremy couldn't tell if they were agreeing with him or doubting that what he'd said was possible.

"It was a very real presence," Jeremy went on. "It was electrifying, really, and it felt very powerful—far more powerful than any of us..." He cast a quick backward glance at Edgar, who was glowering at him from his seat, his arms folded tightly across his chest.

"It is a relief to know that the soul actually exists, and that there is more to us than just blood and...guts." He took another sip of water as he tried to gauge his audience's mood. "I felt very honoured to have been chosen to make contact with it..."

"What did it say?" someone shouted from the audience. A

chorus of cries ensued. "Is there life after death?" "Will you be going to hell?" "Get to the point!"

Jeremy cleared his throat again, and took another deep breath.

"It explained about the importance of soul in our lives, and how an awareness of its purpose can completely transform the way we live."

More murmurs from the crowd.

"It explained how we can get lost along the way if we do not stay connected to the soul, and if we do not follow our hearts and fulfill our dreams, doing the things we were sent here to do and expressing our uniqueness to the world." His voice rose, suddenly strong and confident as he remembered the feeling he had had while the soul spoke to him.

"It showed me how we can heal ourselves, how we can change the way we feel inside by bringing in powerful healing energy and remembering that we are all connected, and all essentially the same."

Another pointed cough came from Edgar behind him, but he carried on regardless.

"It explained how the body gets unhealthy and sick when it is disconnected from the soul, and how many of us live a life devoid of meaning. We have the power to make things happen in our lives, to create magic and to fulfill our enormous potential, way beyond the limits of our negative beliefs, doubts, fears and seemingly mundane existence."

There was a hush now, of a different kind, and he could tell that he had got their attention.

"We have power within us that remains untapped for most of our lives, leaving us empty, unhappy and weighed down by the drudgery and struggle of life. It doesn't need to be this way! The soul showed me what it felt like to be connected to that power, and how I could instantly change my beliefs and the way I feel, so that my experience of life could be completely different. It showed me how I could rise above my fears, my doubts, my limitations, and how I could begin to create a life of tranquility, inspiration and joy."

He looked up at the crowd, his hands resting on the podium before him, his gaze steady.

"The soul's purpose is to help us become aware of our tremendous ability—and responsibility—to positively influence our world, to reawaken our creativity, and to learn a way of conscious living that enables us to experience our ultimate selves. When we connect with the soul and follow its direction, we are taken on a miraculous journey of self-discovery. We are inspired and assisted in fulfilling our dreams, we expand in our capacity to love and be loved, and we constantly go beyond our perceived limits to ever-greater heights of awareness and fulfillment. When we fight against the negative collective beliefs and fears that keep us small, we build emotional muscle and we tap into our individual strengths and gifts. By striving to become fully ourselves, we find fulfillment, we become powerful and we inspire others to do the same."

Jeremy paused for effect, looking up at the crowd again. "It is the ultimate journey."

A smattering of applause broke out, but quickly died away. Jeremy waved a hand in acknowledgement and addressed the crowd again.

"I will be giving classes in meditation and spiritual development to anyone who is interested in learning more," he said. Another murmur rose from the crowd, but no one was more surprised by this statement than Jeremy himself. And he was unable to stop.

"The classes will constitute a complete series designed to help you reawaken your creativity, eliminate negative beliefs and fulfill your dreams. It will—"

"Thank you, Jeremy," Edgar intervened from behind and joined him at the podium. "That's quite enough of the Billy Graham from you, boy," he hissed out of the side of his mouth.

Addressing the crowd, he said, "Ladies and gentlemen, thank you for your attention—"

"If you want to sign up for the course, please see me afterwards!" Jeremy piped up, ignoring Edgar's deadly looks and fairly bouncing up and down on the podium.

"THANK you, Jeremy." Edgar could barely contain his rage. "You may wait for me in my office."

Elated, Jeremy strode confidently off the stage, waving and smiling broadly at his audience as he left. There was only one thing he couldn't figure out. How on earth did Edgar manage to maintain that dazzling smile on his face while spitting venom?

# 22
# Finding fulfillment

"I've been thinking about work," said Jake, leaning on the garden fork. "Trying to decide what to do."

"Mmmmm...?" Sally was down on her hands and knees, planting bulbs in the flowerbed beneath the kitchen window. 'And...?" she looked up at him briefly, brushing a stray strand of hair out of her eyes with the back of her gardening glove.

"I think three months is long enough to convalesce, and I'm ready to take on something new."

"Oh?" Sally turned to face him.

"I think I'd like to become a personal life coach, or some kind of motivational speaker," said Jake. "I want to share my experience with people—inspire them to live more fulfilling and meaningful lives."

"That's wonderful, darling," said Sally, getting up. "But is it practical?" Brushing some grass from her jeans, she looked at him critically. He'd lost a lot of weight since the coronary and had been exercising a lot more over the last six weeks, taking long walks in the woods every morning and gardening with her at the weekends. The warm spring weather had been a godsend, she thought. There was colour in his cheeks and he looked fit, young and downright handsome.

"Depends on what you mean by 'practical'," said Jake. "I want to do something more meaningful—something that I feel passionate and inspired about, that will be rewarding for me and my clients, and that doesn't involve eternal struggle and stress."

"Mmmmm..." said Sally, opening another bag of bulbs. "What brought this on, all of a sudden? I thought you were going to set up your own marketing company."

"I've changed my mind, Sal. I can't go back into marketing." He paused, staring off into the distance. "My heart was never really in it, you know. It just seemed like a good way to make money, but it wasn't me."

He picked up a bulb and turned it over in his hand. "Everything changed with the illness. My values changed. My appreciation of life changed. My capacity for loving, giving, creating, playing, rejoicing... all that changed. Take this bulb, for example."

He held it up and she looked at it skeptically.

"It's a bulb, Jake. You put it in the ground and it grows. Simple."

"Ah, yes," said Jake. "It is simple, isn't it. You water it, give it fertilizer and it becomes a beautiful flower in a few months' time. But put it in the wrong environment—back in the garden shed, say—and nothing will happen. Or, worse still, it will shrivel up and die."

"Why do I feel there is some profound message in here, somewhere?" said Sally, folding her arms across her chest.

"Most of us spend our entire lives in the garden shed, Sal—lying dormant in the dark and never really blooming. We are wasted. We do things that do not nourish us—emotionally or physically—and we wonder why we put on weight, get sick, are unhappy, feel depressed, uninspired, unsuccessful..."

"Yes, but we require a bit more than fertilizer and sunshine, don't we?"

"No, not really," said Jake, taking her hand and leading her down the garden towards the pond.

"You're not just leading me down the garden path, are you?" Sally laughed nervously.

"Love is the fertilizer, Sal; it's our greatest source of nourishment. Without that, we are lost. We can't thrive the way we were designed to. We don't aspire to great things. We lack lustre and sparkle. We can function, but we're not really alive. With the right kind of love in our lives, our hearts are full and we can do anything. And when we follow our hearts, we do what we were born to do."

"And you were born to be a personal coach?"

"I don't know, Sal. All I know is that I need to do something more meaningful, and marketing is not it. The coaching feels right. I've learned a lot about what matters in life and I think I may be able to help others find more fulfillment in their lives. I'll have to get some training, of course, and—"

"See those two sparrows?" said Sally, pointing to the pond.

"Yes," Jake looked at her quizzically.

"They're perfectly happy the way they are. They eat insects, bathe in the pond, sing all morning long and leave when the weather gets bad."

"And...?"

"Some people like things just the way they are, Jake—simple and uncomplicated. They don't necessarily want to change everything."

"Nice try, Sal, but you were the one who wanted me to change, remember? And now that I have, you don't like it. Why is that, do you think?" He looked at her, bemused.

"I *do* like the way you've changed, Jake. It's wonderful. But does *everything* have to change? It feels as if nothing is the same any more and I can't rely on anything staying the same."

"Yes, you can. You can rely on my love and isn't that all that really matters?"

"That could change. You have no way of knowing that it won't." She looked at him defiantly. "People break up all the time, marriages break up, people change their minds."

"Sal, you can't fully love if you're always afraid that it's going to be taken away. At some point, you just have to let go and trust. I learned that when I was on that operating table. Life's not worth living unless we can live it fully. Fear corrodes everything and you never get to see what you could have had. Aren't we worth the gamble, after all we've been through?"

"Maybe. Probably. Just give me a little time to adjust, okay? It's all happening so fast." She smiled, kissed him lightly on the cheek and walked back towards the house.

Jake watched her go. "Don't worry, fellas," he whispered to the sparrows. "Everyone's scared of change—even if they say they want it. She'll come around."

He threw some stones into the pond, reflecting on the ripples that played out to its edges.

"I think I'll order some of her favourite Chinese take-away this evening," he decided, "just so she knows there are some things that never change."

# 23
# Top-secret investigation

Jeremy was about to knock on Lily's office door when she called out to him.

"Let me guess. You've got something on your mind and you want my help."

"Well, actually…" Jeremy smiled sheepishly and sidled into the cramped office.

"Take a seat," said Lily, waving him in the general direction of the wooden chair piled high with papers. She was pouring over some documents on her desk, reading glasses on her nose and a frown bisecting her brow.

"Um, it's okay," said Jeremy. "Should I come back later, when you're not so busy?"

"Ain't gonna happen, not in this lifetime, anyway." Lily took off her glasses, pushed back her chair and looked at him. "What's up?"

"Well, I've been thinking about what the, um, soul said when I met him …it. Something to do with our upbringing and collective beliefs and how that affects our uniqueness and our ability to really be ourselves."

"And?" Lily was getting impatient, eyeing the pile of documents on her desk.

"I have the feeling that it's somehow connected with what happened earlier—with the crisis in the heart department. I think there are some things in there to look at, but I'm not quite sure where to start."

"Turn on that monitor over there," said Lily, pointing to a screen on a shelf behind the door.

Jeremy did so and the screen flickered to life.

"Now click on 'programming'."

"Yeah, okay."

"Now click on EP."

"Um, there's a message. It says 'Top Secret, access denied'."

"Ah, yes. Of course. Just a second." Lily swiveled back to her desk, picked up her cell phone and tapped in a number.

"Crystal? Lily here. I need access to the Early Programming files. Can you give me temporary clearance? I've got Jeremy working on a project down here and he needs some inside info." She paused, waiting as Crystal tapped in some codes at the main console.

"You're in, Lily. Two hours' clearance before automatic lock-out."

"Great. Thanks." Lily put down the phone and turned back to Jeremy.

"Okay, try that again."

Jeremy clicked on 'EP' and another window opened up with several options.

"I've got EP, MPs and BS," said Jeremy, looking totally bewildered. "What IS all this stuff? And why so highly classified?"

"This is the databank for the early programming of the organism and it holds all the records relating to belief systems— that's what BS stands for, among other things."

"And MPs?"

"Well, that refers to his 'missing pieces', which we'll talk about later. Click on EP for now and see what you get."

Jeremy did so.

"It says EP-3 and then there's a whole load of data. What does the 3 stand for?"

"That's when the outside programming kicked in. Up to that point, he was himself. But, at the age of three, the pressure of outside forces became too much and things started to get distorted."

"Things? What kind of things?"

"His beliefs about himself, his internal levels of worthiness, his value, his sense of importance and, most important of all, his 'lovability'—how lovable and deserving he believed himself to be."

"And how does all this relate to the heart failure?" He paused for a second, musing the question. "Hang on, I get it. It's to do with his feelings of low self-worth that pushed him to work too hard, try to prove himself, sabotage his health, all that stuff, right?"

"Yes. Take a look at 'BS: Primary' and see what's listed there."

"Um, let's see…" Jeremy scanned the screen and then clicked on a heading. "Okay, got it. It says Primary BS 'unlovable'."

"That's the main subconscious driver in his life," said Lily. "He doesn't think he's worthy of being loved unconditionally so he tries to earn it and he compensates and compromises himself in lots of ways because he doesn't think he's good enough or lovable enough just as he is."

"But where does this stuff live?" asked Jeremy.

"Most of the time it's in hiding, in the archives. It's not something he's conscious of, otherwise he'd probably try to do something about it. It's buried in these top secret files and only Command Central has access to them."

"But what's the point of that? I mean, that makes no sense. Why doesn't someone access this information and bring it to his attention so that he can work on it and have more love in his life?"

"Well, maybe that will happen now, with your help. Maybe through your work you can enhance his awareness of the soul so that he starts to understand why his heart got so clogged up and why he attracted a partner who has difficulty with intimacy and deep emotional expression."

"Um, I'd need to know the answer to that myself first, though, wouldn't I?"

"The soul works in mysterious ways, Jeremy, as you discovered. It uses our partners as the most powerful reflections of what is going on inside us at the subconscious level. That's a fundamental truth that most people are completely unaware of. As a result, they have one disastrous relationship after another. It's only when they understand that relationships are all about self-discovery and personal empowerment that they can finally take control of their lives."

"So where do we go from here?"

"*We* don't go anywhere," said Lily emphatically. "You're on your own with this one."

"Oh, unlike all the other times, you mean," said Jeremy sarcastically, with a wry smile.

Lily gave him a withering look.

"Hey, I can handle it. You get thrown in the deep end often enough, you learn to swim pretty fast. I'll just have to go back to the soul for some help and inspiration, that's all."

"You'll have to work with Command Central on this, of course," said Lily, turning back to the files on her desk. "You'll need their cooperation for the database and for any re-programming that you might be thinking of doing."

"I can re-program this stuff?"

"If you can figure out the software, yes. And, before you ask, the answer is no, I don't have time to help you with this. Now let me get on with my work."

Jeremy left the office in a daze, his mind buzzing with questions and ideas. He decided to head straight for Command Central; maybe they would see him without an appointment.

# 24
# Intestinal impasse

"Brian, Crystal here. I'm getting a lot of interference on the scanners—a thick fog rolling in from the north, and a ridge of high pressure building up on Fore Head. Not exactly what we need, right now, what with the detox programme just getting under way."

"Yes, Crystal, I know," said Brian. "I've been picking up the same thing myself. What do you suggest we do? I could perhaps send that new guy Arthur in to have a look, if Heather can spare him for a while."

"Yes, good idea," said Crystal. "I'll give him a call."

She reached for her cell phone.

"Arthur? Crystal here. We need you to investigate something for us, please, if you can. There's some interference coming in on our scanners and it looks as if it's originating in the lower digestive tract. Must be because of something His Lordship ate yesterday, but we haven't seen this particular pattern before. Could you get down there and find out what's going on?"

"Certainly, Crystal," said Arthur. "I'm heading south now, and should be there shortly."

★ ★ ★

It was chaos on Highway 22. Traffic was backed up in all directions and nothing was moving. Commuters were getting irate, blowing their horns and shouting obscenities, but to no avail.

At the centre of it all stood a short, wiry young man, who seemed to be the source of the problem. Dressed in long baggy jeans hanging off his hips, a black T-shirt three sizes too large, and a baseball cap on backwards, he was jiving to some inaudible beat from his headphones, seemingly oblivious to the havoc he was causing. Fast approaching down the hard shoulder was Sam, a look of intense fury on his face. He was closely followed by Arthur, who pulled up behind him on his motorbike.

"What the hell is going on?" Sam screamed. "And who are you?"

The youth looked at him insolently, completely unfazed. He continued his rap dance, singing...

*I'm your flavour enhancer*
*I'm the zip in your chip*
*I taste great in your Chinese food*
*I'm trendy, cool and hip...*

"What the...?" Sam was incensed. He lunged for the youth with his fist, but Arthur pulled him back just in time.

*I want a ton of wontons*
*None of those bland ole foods*
*I'll get your brain a spinnin'*
*I'll put a swing in your moods.*

"He came in with that Chinese take-away His Lordship had last night," said Arthur, taking Sam aside. "He's very unpredictable and has caused huge problems in Command Central, as well as in lots of other areas. He'll have to be handled very carefully."

*Just call me Max The Man*
*I'll mix and max your flavour*
*Forget about those side effects*
*Just eat me up and savour...*

"Just tell me how we can get rid of him," said Sam. "That's all I want to know. He left a trail of disaster behind him earlier today in my department, getting everyone hyped up, and I'm ready to lynch the b—"

*I'll tantalize your taste buds*
*You'll become addicted to me*
*I'm your taste sensation*
*Just call me M-S-G.*

"Yes, Sam, I understand," said Arthur. "We need to flush him out, but it will probably take a day or two as we'll have to wait till he's burnt himself out—which he will. He's hyper and never sleeps, so when he finally crashes, we'll get him."

Sam is still fuming, glaring at MSG as he continues to do his ridiculous dance in the middle of the road.

# 25
# Para-military invasion

"Unit 4, are you receiving me?"

"Ten-four, receiving you loud and clear. What is your position?"

"We are a couple of nano-clicks north of ground zero and preparing for the para-drop. Anticipate we will be on the ground at 1900 hours."

"Roger. Confirm arrival and need for back-up when landed."

"Roger that. Over and out."

A flock of parachutes floated down out of the dark sky above Colon County. As they neared the ground, another batch appeared behind them, dropping out of the night as if from nowhere.

Along the northern perimeter of Colon County, para-military units had already infiltrated the area, and were setting up patrol stations at regular intervals.

"Calling all units, calling all units. Ground control here. I need your coordinates and your combat preparedness. Report back ASAP."

"Ground control, this is Unit 5, sir. We are at 54W and 32N on the cellular grid. We are fully operational with system perforators, pathfinders, multi-cell explosives and cellular deprogrammers; with a unit of 400, we're pumped and ready for action, sir."

"Ground control, this is Unit 7 reporting, sir. We are at 46W and 22N on the grid, 300 strong and ready to rock 'n roll with cellular degenerators."

"Ground control, Unit 9 here, sir. We have 580 operatives with two down from the para-drop. Otherwise fully operational with leech feeders, containment mechanisms and anti-organism poppers."

"All units, this is Ground Control. Synchronize your watches and prepare for maximum deployment at 20:00 hours. Your mission is to overwhelm the organism and to set up permanent bases for future operations. Failure to be fully mission-capable will result in termination. Over and out."

★ ★ ★

Jake awoke with a start and sat bolt upright in bed. For a moment, he couldn't remember where he was, the remnants of a ghastly nightmare still swirling around in his brain, and a headache of seismic proportions beginning to throb at his temples. But then he realized he was at Sally's place. He had stayed the night after dinner together by the fire—a Chinese take-away—followed by cuddles and... He groaned as a painful spasm shot through his lower abdomen. As he rolled onto his tummy, Sally stirred and opened her eyes.

"Jake? You okay? It's still early, isn't it?"

"Yes, darling. It's just after 7. Sorry I woke you. I'm not feeling great. That cleanse you put me on must be kicking in."

"Mmmm. It does make you feel awful for a while. All the nasties come out of the woodwork and run rampant in your system. Horrible."

"I feel worse now than when I was supposedly so unhealthy," said Jake, massaging his stomach.

"Meant to," said Sally. "You'll feel better when it's all over, though, so it will be worth it. Honest."

With that, she rolled over and went back to sleep.

Jake stared at her back, wishing he'd never started this whole damn thing, and wishing particularly that he hadn't eaten all that Chinese food last night. It definitely hadn't helped. Come to think of it, should he really have come back down to earth after that coronary...? Throwing back the covers and stumbling heavily from the bed as another spasm shook his bowels, he made a dash for the bathroom.

# 26
# Para panic

"Oh, good lord! I don't believe this. Just when I thought things couldn't possibly get any worse."

Crystal stood transfixed in front of her main monitor, a look of horror on her usually serene face. A scene of dizzying activity confronted her, so frenzied that she could hardly make out what was going on. But she saw enough to get the general idea.

She reached for the phone. "Brian, brace yourself. I've got some very, very bad news. It's the paras. They've infiltrated Colon County, Liver Lay-by, the Central Nervous Station, and it looks as if they are heading this way. I don't know what to do... It's completely overwhelming. How can we possibly strike back and hope to win against this lot? There must be thousands of them..."

"Crystal, get a grip," said Brian. "I'll be right there."

With a click, he was gone, and Crystal remained paralyzed, watching the nightmare unfold on her monitor.

Within minutes, Brian had joined her at the console and was homing in on several key areas to get a better idea of the para-military activity.

"They've set up para-sites all over the place," he said. We're looking at major settlements in Colon County, with a lesser infiltration of the Liver Department, and other minor units heading north, probably to take over Command Central. We're going to have to send out a red alert, and activate all possible Immune Inc. contingents, as well as coming up with other more drastic measures."

He reached for the PA system. "P-Day, P-Day! This is an emergency! We have been invaded by paras and all units must take action immediately. Immune Inc. is in charge. All units must contact Immune Inc. now for their orders, and prepare to counter-attack. The entire organism is at risk." He turned back to Crystal, who was still rooted to the spot in front of her screen.

"Crystal, get me Ace on the line. I need to brief him. Now, Crystal! We haven't a moment to lose."

★ ★ ★

"Okay, teams, let's get organized." Ace stood facing the entire Immune Inc. workforce, planning his strategy. "First, we need to immobilize the main area of infiltration—Colon County. Here." He pointed to a map behind him. "But we must be sure we have the right kind of weaponry to do that. We can't go in there half-cocked, only to discover that they have much more sophisticated artillery—and better intelligence. We need to know exactly what we are up against—"

He was interrupted by his phone ringing. It was Brian, in Command Central.

"Yes, Brian. Tell me what you've got."

"Ace, I've just done some quick research and here's what I have so far. There seem to be three main para-sites and, if I'm right, they are not quite as lethal as we first thought. That's the good news. The bad news is that they proliferate rapidly and will expand hugely in numbers if we don't get in there fast.

"So, who are we dealing with, Brian? I need to get my teams activated straight away."

"Right. Well, all three seem to have similar modus operandi. They can perforate all our structures and infiltrate most organs. They are single-celled and agile, with lots of experience in weakening an entire organism. They locate their bases in Colon County and branch out from there, scavenging, feeding off our resources, and dumping waste along the way, making the system even more toxic and causing spasmodic flushing of the system."

"What's their weak point, Brian?" said Ace. "We need to know how to bring them down."

"There are certain substances that knock them out, but we don't have all of them in stock. We'll have to get them ordered in, and that's the problem…"

"What are they, Brian? And what can we do in the meantime?"

"There's a grapefruit-seed extract, black walnut extract, a herb called wormwood, cloves, and several other potent natural things that tend to kill them off when used for several months. There are other chemicals that will do the same job, and faster, but they're much harder on the system. So, for the moment, all we can do is try to surround them, and contain them until the message gets through on the outside that some ammunition needs to be sent in."

"Okay, Brian. We'll take it from here. I'll update you later."

Ace turned back to his men.

"We're going to have to go in with what we've got and do the best we can to surround and contain the enemy," he said. "We need to blunt their edge until more ammo gets shipped in and we have the means to knock the stuffing out of them. In the meantime, I want three teams to go straight to Colon County and begin the offensive. Stay in touch by radio, and we'll send in another team to do some post-strike reconnaissance. Any questions?"

"I've heard that this lot are particularly vicious and nasty, sir," said one of his team leaders. "Do we have any more intelligence on them and their MO that might help us stay ahead of the game?"

"Well, they are very fast and nimble, by all accounts," said Ace. "They also tend to use their sheer numbers rather than their intelligence to overcome their opponents. So perhaps we can catch them out in terms of tactics, even if we are slightly deficient in numbers and ammo. Any more suggestions before we head out?"

He looked around the room.

"Sir, if they are heading north towards Command Central, I think we should try to intercept them before they get into the Heartland."

"Yes," said Ace. "Indeed. But now that they have infiltrated Colon County and penetrated the Alimentary Canal, they'll be travelling north via the Blood Stream, which means they could be anywhere."

"Sir, if I may suggest something." Another operative raised his hand.

"Yes, Agent Luke O'Cyte?"

"We could deploy our transponder equipment in the areas already infiltrated, to identify friend from foe. Maybe this would be useful as a quick recce before we deploy our forces."

"Excellent suggestion. I'd like you and your team to get on that right away. Once we have an idea of their whereabouts, we'll send out teams and have them surrounded by early morning. Keep me posted on your progress. I'll be in Command Central if anyone needs me."

★ ★ ★

Unit 4's commander was getting impatient. His men had plundered and pillaged all night but they hadn't made any significant progress in their mission. He needed to see some real military action. After summoning his unit to the para-site headquarters, he told them what he wanted to do.

"Men, we need to get tough with these natives. We're not having enough of a negative impact and we need to up the ante. I want to see more cellular degeneration, more perforation of cellular walls, and leakage of essential nutrients. Go for their weak spots—women and children. Be merciless. I won't have any namby-pamby softies in my unit. DO YOU READ ME?" He paced back and forth in front of his men, his eyes fixing them with his intense stare. They were getting the message. Failure was not an option. "Spread out. Teams of 50. Go for any station that's manned, eh, so to speak, by a woman. Be brutal. I want aggression, torture, degradation, debasement, humiliation— your entire arsenal put to best effect. Only when we've weakened certain core areas can we begin to take control. And we're a long way from that yet. So let's see some action. Report back at 06:00."

There was a deafening noise of chairs scraping back, rifles being hefted onto shoulders, and big heavy army boots heading for the door as some 500 operatives prepared to deploy. At the edge of camp, a large river flowed rapidly by. Along its banks, several boats were moored, bobbing up and down. The paras split into groups, filed into the boats and headed upstream in a roar of powerful motors and churning wakes.

Five hundred metres upstream, the lead boat signaled to the others and turned left into a tributary marked Liver Station.

★ ★ ★

As usual, Lily had far too much to do. She and Oliver had worked late into the night, managing the toxic backlog and strategizing on their defence against the latest assault on the system. She was exhausted, and the only thing she wanted to do now was sleep and maybe—

"Up against the wall! Move it!"

Her hands were yanked roughly behind her back, and she was shoved hard against the wall.

Suddenly, paras were swarming all over the place, pulling out the files from her filing cabinets, spraying graffiti on the walls, overturning furniture, smashing the windows, and ripping the doors from their hinges.

# 27
# Healing begins

"There is an intestinal problem," the healer said, placing her hand on his abdomen. "There is an invasion of unfriendly organisms in your system, and you will need to take some strong remedies to get rid of them."

Jake was lying on his back on an examining table, staring up at the wise old face of the healer as her hands moved over his body.

"What kind of organisms?" he asked. "What kind of remedies?"

"Nothing too serious. Some single-celled parasites. But, if left untreated, they can create havoc."

She reached behind her to an assortment of bottles on a table.

"Take three of these on an empty stomach in the morning, for three weeks, then come back to see me." She handed him a glass bottle filled with dark-brown capsules.

"They can be stubborn, these organisms, and we need to make sure they're completely wiped out. But don't be surprised if you feel a bit worse for a while as they die off. It's a good sign and you just need to persist and drink lots of pure water to flush them out of your system."

"What are they?" Jake examined the bottle.

"Capsules of goldenseal—a potent natural herb used to kill off certain organisms. They're also a natural anti-bacterial so they will help clean up any other unfriendly flora in there."

"I'll take them," Jake said, getting up off the table. "I'm determined to get healthy."

"Well, then, there's one more thing," said the healer, staying him with her hand.

"Oh?" said Jake.

"Invading organisms, such as parasites, are often a sign that one's boundaries are weak, so there may be some work to do there."

"I don't know what you mean," Jake said. "What kind of boundaries?"

"Personal ones," said the healer. "Very often related to what you want to do with your life, which may be restricted in some way because of pressure from a loved one, for example. There is something you want to do, but you are having difficulty accomplishing it. Does this sound familiar?"

"Yes, it does," said Jake. He was thoughtful for a moment. "Do you have any idea what that 'something' might be? I'm not sure I'm on the right track."

"You are sure, and you are on the right track. What brought you here?"

"I heard about your through a friend, and something told me I needed to see you."

"You knew what you needed, and you know where to go from here. You must simply make the decision and go for it wholeheartedly. The universe will move with you, supporting you in ways you could not have imagined. You are a teacher and an inspiration for others. That is your calling. Get rid of these invaders in your system, build strength in your conviction, and follow your heart. Do not let others hold you back. Do this and your life and health will be strong."

Jake felt a wave of gratitude wash over him. And something more—a sense of some kind of connection with the bigger picture, and an acute awareness of his unique place within it.

"Stay in touch," said the healer, taking his hand warmly in hers.

"Yes, I'll call you," said Jake.

"Not with me," said the healer. "With your self."

# 28
# Covert immunity

"Ace, it looks as if we've got the ammo we need," said Brian. "Just got word that some powerful anti-para material is entering the system. Stand by for deployment."

"Good news, Brian. And not a moment too soon. Lily has been taken hostage and we haven't been able to break their ranks to reach her. We've been receiving emergency calls for help from her unit and we need to get in there fast."

"It's on its way," said Brian. "Stay in position on the outskirts of Liver Valley and be ready. It should be with you shortly."

Ace turned back to his men.

"Right, men. This is it. Ammo is on the way. When it gets here, I want you to fully surround the perimeter and go in full blast. We need to stun them with this stuff so we can overcome their numbers more easily."

Even as he spoke, they could hear something rushing down the Alimentary Canal towards them, preceded by a strange golden hue.

"What is that?" said Ace, mesmerized by the sight.

The golden light grew stronger, and suddenly a truckload of about 20 squat men emerged from the canal. Dressed in metallic, golden-coloured suits, they were fit and muscled, armed to the teeth with strange weapons that Ace had never seen before.

"Eh, welcome," he said. "You must be…."

"We're the Goldenseal Team," said the team leader, emerging from the vehicle. "Where's the action? We'll get straight to work."

"It's in Liver Valley, just west of here," said Ace. "But we'll need to brief you…"

"No need," said the leader. "We know what to do. Ready guys?"

"Just a second," said Ace. "What exactly are you going to use to wipe this lot out? They're not your average everyday bacteria, you know."

"And we're not your average everyday annihilation team," the team leader retorted. "We'll be using special high-potency organisms to blast this lot into outer space. They'll be no match for us. We'll take out the most threatening contingent in Liver Valley now, and then spread out into the further reaches of the system to track down the rest of them over the next few days. They'll be gone within the week."

"Okay. Right," said Ace, uncertainly. "Very impressive. What can we do?"

"Nothing. Just stay out of the way and stand by to help clear up the mess afterwards. There will be a lot of toxic waste to get rid of." He turned back to his team.

"Men, let's go deal with these vermin."

# 29
# Inside info

"Hi. I'm Jake Jordan. I have a 2 o'clock appointment with Victoria Granger. But I'm a little early…"

"Oh, yes, Mr Jordan. Victoria is ready, actually. Just go down the corridor and you'll see her office, first on the left."

"Right. Thanks."

Jake was just about to do so when a petite, 30-something redhead came to meet him.

"Jake, I'm Vicky." She extended her hand and grasped his warmly. "Come this way. I'm glad you're early. My last client had to cancel at the last minute."

He followed her into a sunlit room containing a bookcase, a small desk and a massage table covered with a soft, white blanket.

"Take a seat, Jake, please." Victoria gestured to the chair on the other side of her desk as she sat down opposite him. "Now, I just need to get a few details from you before we start. How did you find out about me, by the way?"

"I heard about you through a healer I consulted a while ago…"

"Ah, yes. That would be Angela. Lovely woman. Now… I'll need you to just fill out your medical details and sign this disclaimer form, then we can get started." She passed him a clipboard and a pen. "I'm not sure how much Angela told you about my work. Do you have any questions?"

"She didn't say much, only that you were very good and she felt it would be helpful for me to see you. So I really have no idea what you do."

"Well, some people refer to me as a bio-kinesiologist, but I prefer to think of myself as an inspirational coach," said Vicky, smiling. "There is a technique in kinesiology called muscle-testing, which was developed by a chiropractor as a way of finding out what is going on inside the body, and I use that to obtain all kinds of information. You'll get to see how that works in a minute. However, I take a slightly more integrated approach than traditional kinesiologists, looking at the subconscious programming, relationship dynamics, the emotional functions of the various organs, and whatever may be stopping you from being your true self." She paused to let that sink in. "I can use this same technique to talk to the body to find out what it needs in the way of nutrients, supplements or anything else that will help it to stay healthy and balanced."

"Sounds great," Jake handed her back the clipboard. "Can this technique also help with one's life purpose, career, that kind of thing?"

"Yes, that too," said Vicky, getting up and moving over to the massage table. "It's all about you being yourself, getting the most out of life and letting go of old habits or beliefs that stop you from being everything you have the potential to be." She gestured for Jake to lie down on the table. "Of course, there's some work involved, but you wouldn't be here unless you wanted to make some changes, right?"

"Yes, absolutely," said Jake, looking a little uncertainly up at the white ceiling.

Vicky patted Jake's arm and smiled at him. "Just relax. I'm going to be using your arm to muscle-test, raising it like this at about a 45-degree angle and applying some gentle pressure. I want you to hold it in place—just enough to stop me pushing it back down. That's right. Perfect. I'm going to be asking some questions of the body, silently; if I press on your arm and the answer is no, you'll feel your arm go weak. If the answer is yes, the arm will remain strong. When I've obtained all the information I need, I'll fill you in. In the meantime, just close your eyes and relax."

★ ★ ★

"Attention, please! This is Command Central, calling all directors. Please assemble in the main communications hall immediately. Your input is urgently required. Attention, please…"

"I wonder what that's about," said Billy Gallbladder, pulling on his coat and picking up his briefcase on his way out the door.

"Gilly, please keep an eye on things here while I'm gone. Any decisions to be made can wait till I get back." He smiled at his secretary and hurried off.

He took the tube north and got out at the Cerebral Cortex Auditorium. He arrived to find the hall rapidly filling up. There was a sense of excited anticipation in the air.

"Settle down, everyone, please." Brian stood at the top of the hall and gestured for some last-minute arrivals to be seated.

"This is a rather exceptional meeting." He cleared his throat, his expression serious. "Unprecedented, you might say."

There was a murmur from the crowd.

"We have, as it were, a 'hot line' to the outside world, giving us a rare opportunity to communicate our needs and explain the conditions in our respective departments."

There was an agitated buzz from the hall.

"Quiet, please. Let me explain. His Lordship is consulting a sort of medium, as far as I can tell—someone who has the ability to communicate directly with our various departments and to hear what we have to say. This is the opportunity we have been waiting for, and it could be an important turning point."

He turned to a small radio-like apparatus on the table beside him.

"I have here a two-way radio transmitter so that we can tune in to what is going on and, hopefully, get good enough reception to catch everything that's being said. Transmission began a few moments ago, so hopefully we haven't missed too much. Please try to be quiet as I adjust the frequency."

He twiddled the tuning knob on the radio and loud static filled the hall. Then, suddenly, a voice came clearly and audibly over the airwaves.

"Does the heart need help?"

Brian gesticulated urgently to Heather.

"Answer her, Heather, please. Go ahead. Quickly."

Heather, flustered, walked quickly up to the radio and leaned towards it.

"Yes," she said. "Yes, we do, we…"

126

Brian interjected quickly. "Heather, sorry, I forgot to say, we can only give yes or no answers. I don't know why. It's some sort of special system that I don't quite understand. So just wait for the next question."

"Okay, right." Heather looked expectantly at the radio.

"Is the problem nutritional?"

"Yes, partially… I mean, yes."

"Are there any emotional factors involved?"

"Yes, definitely."

"Spiritual?"

"Yes." Heather was starting to get exasperated. Where was this going?

"Good," said the voice. "Now I'm starting to get the picture. I'm going to run through some options here and I want you to let me know when I touch on something relevant. Then just give me a yes."

Heather waited.

"Fat intake—quantity, quality…"

"Yes to both," said Heather.

"Too much stress, more exercise required, need for supplements…."

"Yes to supplements."

"Vitamins…"

"Yes."

"Vitamin A, beta-carotene, B complex…"

"Yes to B complex."

"C, D, E. Minerals..."

"Yes to minerals."

"Chromium, iron, iodine, calcium, magnesium…"

"Yes to magnesium."

"…zinc, phosphorous, potassium, selenium…"

"Yes to selenium."

"Trace minerals…"

"Yes."

"Any others?"

"Yes."

"Let's see… CoQ10, enzymes…"

"Yes! Yes to enzymes."

"…lecithin…"

"Yes, lots."

"Anything else in the way of supplements?"

"No."

"Right," said the voice. "Let me just make some notes and then we'll look at some specific foods, and the emotional aspects involved."

Brian turned to Heather.

"This could take a while. I need to get back upstairs. Just keep going till you've answered all her questions. And if there's anything important she's overlooked, try to get that message across."

He turned back to the hall.

"Only the main departments are going to be consulted, so only directors with grievances or special requests need stay. Everyone else can get back to work, but keep your cell phones handy in case your input is needed."

Brian turned back to Heather who was once again talking into the radio.

"…yes to low self-esteem, weak personal boundaries, and indecision due to fear of failure…"

"Blimey," said Sam, who was sitting in the front row, next to Pete Pancreas. "She's really going for it, isn't she?"

"Well, it's a make-or-break scenario, I think, Sam. Glad she mentioned those enzymes, though. That will make my job much easier."

"Yeah. Mine, too, actually. But I hope we get our say, as well."

He paused, lost in thought.

"I wonder if she'll get to talk to the soul, like that chap Jeremy did… That could put a whole new spin on things."

★ ★ ★

"Well, Jake, we've got some interesting information for you to work with, don't you think?" Vicky looked at him as he sat up slowly and swung his legs over the side of the table.

"It's all a bit much to take in," said Jake. "In fact, I'm feeling a bit woozy."

"Perfectly normal. There's a lot happening on the inside that you may not be aware of consciously. There are going to be big changes in your life, and it will feel as if things are shifting on all levels, which can sometimes be a bit unsettling. Not everyone will want these changes."

She looked at him meaningfully.

"Yes, I understand."

"But they are inevitable. And your health and well-being will improve greatly as a result."

Vicky sat down at her desk again and began making some notes for Jake.

"You know, Jake, many people resist change for fear that their lives will fall apart, or that they'll lose whatever it is they're afraid of losing—a partner, a convenient marriage, any kind of dynamic that seems to meet their needs. But very often not changing results in far greater loss or upheaval—and it is all the more painful when it occurs at the last stage of an inevitable outcome."

"Yes, I do know what you mean. I've had a few of those myself, in the past. Wake-up calls, I think they're called."

Jake stood up slowly, running his fingers through his hair.

"Wow." He steadied himself against the side of the table. "I feel as if I've just run a marathon."

"You must rest. Don't underestimate what has happened here today. You're going to be processing a lot of emotions and old programming as they come to the surface to be cleared out. Changes are already under way and if you do these exercises…" She passed him a sheet of paper. "…take the supplements and work on those emotional issues I mentioned, you'll find that things will have shifted considerably within about a month."

She walked him to the door.

"And don't forget: filling in those 'missing pieces' I talked about will bring about the most powerful transformations for you—personally as well as professionally. Don't allow any self-doubts to creep in. You have everything you need to succeed."

# 30
# Bummed out and burned out

"I don't think I've ever felt so depressed. I'm tired, I'm irritable, I don't sleep well, I wake up at night with my heart pounding, I have night sweats, anxiety and nightmares, and I feel exhausted most of the time. I'm overworked and can't keep up with the demand for all the hormones I'm supposed to be supplying to the rest of the system. And I feel as if there is nothing happening in my life, as if I'm on hold…"

Andrew Adrenal lay listlessly on the couch, looking vacantly up at the ceiling.

"How long have you felt like this, Andrew?"

Dr Medulla sat beside him on a chair, clipboard on her knee.

"Oh, I don't know… months, years. It just sort of crept up on me, and now I feel pretty crummy most of the time. I have no motivation to work, my orders and inventories are behind schedule, and I feel I have no control over anything or even any desire to fix things. I just feel defeated and—"

"Yes, well, that's why you're here. We're going to look at all this." Dr Medulla spoke soothingly while taking notes.

"I've got the results of your tests here, and they confirm that you're suffering from chronic exhaustion, with corticol and other hormonal imbalances, which I'll explain in a moment. I'm assuming you've had fairly sustained stress over the past few years, if the general chaos around here recently has been anything to go by?"

"Yes," said Andrew. "Far too much stress, and no one to help relieve it. And there has been so much going on in my personal life, too. Lots of change, relationship challenges and no real new direction…"

"Andrew, what you have is very common, nowadays, but none the less serious. It's a depletion that can be caused by a number of different stressors—too much work, emotional problems, bad digestion, not enough sleep, too much sugar in the diet, too much caffeine, etc. But it can be reversed, if you're willing to follow a fairly specific programme."

She looked at him.

"Well, yes, of course. Anything to feel normal again," said Andrew. "As long as I can get some time off…"

"First, you must remove the stressors in your life—somehow handle or resolve them so that they do not continue to wear you down. Can you do that?"

"Well…"

"If your life depended on it?"

"Yes. I suppose so…"

"Good. Want to talk about them?"

"No, thanks. I can handle them."

"Fine, but please bear in mind that you have very specific characteristics that make you more susceptible to exhaustion than most, so you must watch out for those. You have a very finely tuned fight-or-flight mechanism. Do you know what that is?"

"Yes, I think so. It's what our ancestors did to stay safe, isn't it? They either attacked their predator or ran away to avoid being eaten. Right?"

"Yes, that's exactly it. However, you still have this primal mechanism built into you. So when you are faced with stress, the healthy thing to do would be to either address the source of the stress immediately, or move away from it and get some intensive exercise to defuse the charge caused by whatever is stressing you."

"Good theory," said Andrew, "but not that easy to do when you're in a meeting, say, or faced with a tight deadline for something very important. I can't exactly get up and sprint around the boardroom table, can I?"

"Well, that would be the best option. But if you can't do it in the moment, do it as soon afterwards as possible. The important thing is for the stress to be defused so that it does not build up and cause a problem. Think you can give that a try over the next few weeks?"

"I'll try, but no guarantees."

"Good. Secondly, you must try to get your colleagues to change their working hours so that fewer demands are placed on you. Your most important shift is between 10pm and 1am, which is when you and your team do your best work and make the most repairs on the organism. You need this time to work in peace, without interruption. If you do this, you'll naturally find yourself getting into gear again at about 6am, before everyone else starts their day. This way, you can more easily manage your hormonal deliveries and dispatch—particularly that all-important corticol I mentioned earlier. As you know, that's fundamental to your work so you need to be sure that the supply meets the demand. Any shortfall or imbalance there can lead to all kinds of problems in the organism—insulin insensitivity, exhaustion, depression, infections, fluid retention, osteoporosis, high blood pressure..."

"I'm worn out just thinking about it."

"Andrew, you must not underestimate the emotional impact on your system. Because of the amount of stress you have to handle in your work, when you get depleted, you get discouraged and then you become caught up in a vicious cycle that makes it very hard to motivate yourself to do what it takes to get well. The positive counterpart to discouragement is excitement and that is what you need in order to stimulate your entire department and generate the energy you need to bring things back into balance. So let's work on that, okay?"

# 31
# Detox denial

"Okay, everyone, this is the last part of our detox programme and today we're going to be working on our emotions."

Loud groans went up from the room.

"Now that's exactly the problem, right there," said Dietrich, waving a finger at the group in front of him. "The emotional part is always pushed aside as unimportant, yet we create havoc if we don't take care of our emotions and learn how to deal with them in healthy ways. And men are particularly guilty of this."

He looked pointedly at the 20 participants, over half of whom were men.

"Now, you each have some very specific emotions to deal with in your respective lines of work. You may be aware of them but I've made a list here of what they are, just in case…" He picked up a pile of paper and handed it to Kyla who was sitting nearest him. "Pass these around, please, Kyla."

He turned back to the group.

"As you can see, you all have some homework to do. The emotions you are dealing with have a very specific and deleterious impact on your work and your health. So I want to go around the table and have each of you read out the section on your department and tell me what you can do to improve things. Sam, let's start with you."

"Um, right, okay. Says here, 'Fears and anxieties, which particularly affect acid levels. People who have chronic acid problems tend to have a nervous constitution and suffer from gas and heartburn'. Doesn't really sound like me, though, does it? I mean, I get a bit worked up, sometimes, but—"

"Are you kidding?" Oliver was indignant. "You're forever worrying about things and going on at us about things not being done right."

"Sam, let's look at how you might be more relaxed, in general," said Dietrich. "Can you identify the kind of thing that normally annoys you?"

"Well, comments like that, for a start." Sam glared at Oliver. "Nothing but criticism, that's what really gets to me. I mean, I have huge responsibilities, and a lot of stress, and I really don't feel as if I get a lot of… a lot of support most of the time."

Sam cleared his throat and stared fixedly at his notebook in front of him, refusing to look Dietrich in the eye.

"Okay, Sam. Thank you. We can certainly appreciate how you're feeling. And it's good to get it off your chest. What would it take for you to feel more supported?"

"Well, I can't remember the last time I had any positive encouragement. Some of that would go a long way towards making me feel a bit more… well, a bit more… appreciated. My department plays a crucial role in this organism and we are the first ones to take any meaningful action in the breakdown of foods. So much depends on us. If we don't do our job properly, everyone else further down the line suffers. So…more appreciation for what we do and for who we are would certainly help."

Sam was quite red in the face and he returned to studying his notebook.

"Excellent," said Dietrich. "I hope you've all taken note of what Sam said and will think of it when you're working with him in future. Now, moving along… Andrew, you're next."

"Right, okay. 'Exhaustion, worry, lacking in courage; feeling as if people are slowly draining my energy and not wanting to talk about my condition,' it says here. Well, the last bit is right, anyway. I don't really see any point in talking about it. Never changes anything, does it, so why bother?"

He looked defiantly at Dietrich.

"Andrew, I'm afraid that kind of attitude won't help. It's precisely by expressing your concerns that we gain a better understanding of what's required in order for things to function better. If you keep it all inside, then things can go seriously wrong and everyone suffers ultimately, including you, of course.

So, please, indulge me with some details."

"Well, you know, I'm already getting help with this. I'm actually seeing someone professionally, so I don't need to do this here."

Dietrich sighed heavily and fixed him with an unwavering stare.

"Okay, okay. If you must know, I feel utterly worn out and have no sense of pride in my work the way I used to. I feel conflicted all the time, constantly pulled in different directions by competing priorities. I'm fighting a losing battle, with no sense of accomplishment. It leaves me feeling very drained at the end of the day and, frankly, not really caring whether the organism lives or dies. There. You asked for it."

"That's fine, Andrew. There's nothing wrong with feeling that way. But let's see how we can help you. What would it take for you to feel better in yourself and in your work?"

"Ha. A miracle. I'd need help from the outside. I'd need.... Look, I really don't want to talk about it any more."

"Andrew, can't you see that you're just proving the point? One of your classic symptoms is not wanting to talk about your condition. Now, please, go on."

Andrew sighed dramatically.

"I need to be powerful in my work. I need to be able to stand my ground when stress levels go off the scale, to hold my space in the face of pressure, and to say no, when necessary. I need to feel that I am powerful enough to resolve all the conflicts that I have to deal with, and to feel proud of the way I've handled things."

"So what can we do to help? What do you need?"

"I need lots more nutrients, to start with—B complex, minerals... Plus, I need for His Lordship to avoid alcohol, caffeine and tobacco, which are all highly toxic for my department, especially when we're so run down. But how likely is that? See? No point..." He raised his arms in defeat and then folded them across his chest.

"Andrew, as you know, a lot of this information has been

brought to His Lordship's attention now, so it's very likely that you'll get what you want. What else do you need?"

"He'd have to give up bad fats, fried foods, ham, pork, highly processed foods, red meats, sugar, white flour… all of which put us under unnecessary stress. He'd have to eat plenty of fresh fruit and vegetables, particularly green leafy ones, and, well, you know… a healthy diet. He'd also have to be sure to avoid stressful situations and get moderate exercise every day. He'd also have to start making strong, healthy boundaries in his relationships and saying no to unhealthy compromises. In short, he'd have to be a bit of a saint. Like I said, not likely t—"

"Well, Andrew, some of this is already happening, you know. It's just that you've been battling with all this for so long that you've given up hope of ever having a quiet life. And maybe you haven't even noticed that things have changed. But His Lordship is now exercising daily and he's given up that job that caused such stress in the past. He's also eating much better, so we just need to press home the need to reduce the caffeine intake and fine-tune a few other dietary aspects. Which leaves the emotional aspect. What do you need there in order to feel better?"

"I need to know that I'm good enough. I need to have my capacities recognized and I need to have my authority respected. When I'm faced with pressure and I make certain decisions, I need them to be respected. Old habits die hard, though, so I'm not too optimistic about this…"

"Well, start being optimistic, Andrew, because that in itself will help. We all need to give each other—and ourselves— positive encouragement and recognition for who we are. So no more putting yourself down, please."

"Yeah, that's *our* job," quipped Oliver, with an impish grin.

Dietrich glared at him. "Not funny, Oliver. As I was saying, Andrew, get the rest you need, now that things have quietened down a bit, and open up to the possibility that things are actually improving—because they are."

Dietrich consulted his notes.

"Okay, let's take a break. I want you each to think about the emotions on your list and to come up with a positive affirmation to re-program your systems."

This was greeted with another loud groan.

"Affirmations? That's namby-pamby, New Age stuff," said Kyla Kidney. "What earthly good is that going to do us?"

"Affirmations are very powerful. They are designed to help you change your minds about yourselves. And 'mind over matter' is precisely what this is all about. Mind creates matter. Think about how many negative thoughts you have every day, every minute. And if those thoughts create matter, imagine just how much havoc you must all be creating."

He waved away further objections.

"You don't have to take my word for it. Spend one week focusing on negative thoughts and see how you feel. Then do one week filled with positive thoughts and observe the changes. Not that you'll find that easy… since most of you have proved yourselves to be more than a little negative. And, of course, it's far easier to blame others for what happens to us in life than to take responsibility for things ourselves and realize that we actually do have some control over our circumstances. Rather childish, that, and a waste of precious life, I'd say. Any other questions?"

There were none.

"Back here in half an hour. And please bring your self-responsibility with you."

# 32
# Wasteland below the waistband

The streets of the Lower Alimentary Canal were deserted. The cool, gray light of 4am cast eerie shadows on the round, corrugated walls. A single dead cell rolled slowly along the street, like the dry husk of a sea urchin. Fragments of old fecal matter could be seen encrusted in the walls, aged and hardened, and unlikely to be removed by anything less than a stick of dynamite. The air was desert-dry and hot, the stuffiness intensified by every parched breath that passed through. The walls looked old, like the skin of a dehydrated 80-year-old woman who had never heard of moisturizing cream. A still, expectant heaviness hung in the air, as if the whole Alimentary Canal were a vast sponge waiting for moisture to swell it into action once again. A closed-circuit TV camera turned jerkily on its rusty mounts, creaking crankily as it took in the scene. The lens was coated with fecal particles and grime from years of neglect, and it was no longer getting the full picture. A sudden gust of fetid wind raised eddies of dust along the street, lending it the sorry, neglected air of an abandoned set for an old Hollywood western.

As the early-dawn light began to filter down into the bowels of the organism, and distant rumblings reverberated throughout the system, a lone figure could be seen wending its way slowly along the Canal. He carried a torch and was peering closely at the walls on both sides.

"Disgusting," Arthur Artery muttered to himself. "A filthy, unhygienic dump. Looks as if it hasn't been cared for in decades. And they wonder why there's congestion in the works… How can any nutrients survive in such an unkempt, barren wasteland?"

He scanned the walls, finally zeroing in on the camera.

"What the…?" He pulled a small bottle of liquid and a rag out of the pocket of his rucksack. "How the heck can they monitor conditions if they don't even maintain the surveillance equipment?"

He squirted some liquid onto the cloth and rubbed the lens. The cloth came away filthy and he repeated the process, finally seeing some shiny clear glass.

"There. That's better." He put the cloth and bottle back in his rucksack. "If they just had some simple procedures here they wouldn't even need me."

Arthur continued along the Canal, occasionally taking samples of matter from the walls and placing them carefully in zippered bags that he then dropped into the small canvas knapsack on his back. He glanced at his watch and picked up the pace. It would soon be time for breakfast and he'd have to be finished and out of here by then, if he valued his health.

# 33
# Lymphomaniacs

Nicholas Nodes was having difficulty thinking clearly. He scratched his head and got up from his desk to stretch his legs. It was amazing how exhausting staring at a monitor could be, and he wasn't sure he was ever going to figure out how to motivate his sluggish unit to get its act together. He was about to reach for a coffee from the machine in the corner of his office, when there was a timid knock on the door. He looked up. A young man and woman stood in the doorway, each clasping a pile of books and folders.

"Yes? Can I help you?"

"Well, yes, we hope so," said the young man. "My name is Oscar O'Lymphus and this is…"

"I'm Ana Tomi," said the young woman, who looked as if she was no more than 16.

"We're students, and we were hoping you could help us out with some information," said Oscar. "I'm writing my doctorate thesis on a particular aspect of the lymphatic system and Ana is doing general studies. We—"

"Look, I really don't have time for this," said Nicholas, impatiently running his hands through his tousled hair. "I'm extremely busy and—"

"We'll be really quick," said Ana. "If you could just show us around your unit, then we'll be out of your, eh, hair."

"It will have to be very quick, then," said Nicholas ungraciously, grabbing his cell phone from his desk and ushering them out the door.

"I'll give you the tour of this unit only; for the rest of the department, you'll have to see the other unit heads."

"Who would they be?" Oscar whipped out his pen, ready to jot down their names.

"Lindy Lymph is the departmental head, so you should see her. Then the other unit heads are Sophie Spleen, Tessa Thymus, Taddy Tonsils, Mandy Bone Marrow and Axel Appendix, although he doesn't have much to do, these days. There's a lot of debate about just how useful his unit is, but he's never really proved himself to be essential to the department. Bit of a dead-end area, in my opinion, but there you go…"

Nicholas was walking swiftly down the corridor, the two students in hot pursuit, Oscar scribbling as they went.

They continued down a long corridor, turned a corner and arrived in an open-plan area that was alive with activity. Dozens of oval-shaped bodies were moving around but it seemed to Ana that they were moving in slow motion.

"What are these?" she asked, gesturing.

"These are some of the hundred or so lymph nodes that make up my unit," said Nicholas, sighing heavily.

"You don't sound too happy about that," observed Oscar.

"Well, I'm not. In fact, I'm pissed off with them all at the moment," said Nicholas, suddenly feeling very much so. "I've got nerds for nodes and I'm sick and tired of trying to get them to clear up all this clutter that they live in."

He gestured to the mounds of what looked like soft tissue lying in clumps all over the place.

"What are they supposed to do?" asked Oscar.

"They're supposed to act as barriers to infection by filtering out and destroying toxins and germs. But look at all this stuff lying around. It's nothing but toxins and germs."

"So, how can you clear things up?"

"For the unit to function properly—the whole department, in fact—the nodes need to be able to dump their infection-fighting cells quickly into the blood stream. But they've been far too sluggish recently because of a minor infection, which causes them to swell up and then things get congested."

"Actually, I have a theory about this," Oscar interjected. "It's the subject of my thesis, in fact."

"Great. Just what I need. Another theory," said Nicholas

impatiently, but seeing Oscar's crestfallen expression, he relented. "Let's hear it, then."

Oscar cleared his throat and shuffled his books nervously before continuing.

"What I've observed is that the whole lymphatic system is designed to detoxify the system, right?"

"Yes, that is what we do, here, you know." Nicholas looked pointedly at his watch.

"Well, at a physical level, yes. But what causes these toxins to build up in the first place?" Nicholas opened his mouth to reply but Oscar rushed on, warming to his subject. "I believe that the organism can not keep itself free of toxins if it does not have a full understanding of how it works and who it is."

"Look, I appreciate your theories, but I think we all have a fairly good idea down here of how things work. Now, if you'll excuse me…"

Nicholas turned to go, but Oscar continued.

"Yes, we do, I know, but what about His Lordship? That's where the problem is. If he doesn't understand who he is and how all his different departments function, how can he deal with difficult situations? And if he can't do that, he has to find some way of blocking out the pain or discomfort that results. So he eats or drinks or smokes, and then things get congested. Emotions get blocked and you end up having to deal with them here." He gestured at all the sluggish nodes and the mounds of tissue around them.

"Well, that's very interesting," said Nicholas, edging his way back along the corridor. "Now I really must be getting back…"

"But Mr, eh, Nodes… wait, please." Oscar hurried after him. "Might I suggest that the problem you are facing at the moment could be resolved if you applied this theory?"

"And how exactly might I do that?" Nicholas looked over his shoulder but kept walking.

"I really believe that if you promoted a deeper understanding of the organism and tried to explain some of the mystery—at the emotional and spiritual levels—then things would really improve."

"Emotional and spiritual stuff… that's not my job. I'm hired to supervise this lot and make sure they keep the place clean."

"But it's not working, is it?" Oscar ran around in front of Nicholas and blocked his path. "You're left with a bunch of lymphomaniacs who—"

"A bunch of *what*?" Nicholas was obviously reaching the end of his rope.

"Well, see, that's all part of my theory. Lymphomaniacs are what you get when you lose your sense of self. You don't know who you are or how to reject toxic stuff so that things function perfectly, inside and out. We all grow up thinking we have to take on things that are bad for us, in order to be accepted and liked by others. That's what you're dealing with here." He gestured back towards the chamber of listless nodes. "That's why they can't get their act together. They don't know how to process all this toxic stuff because they don't really understand who they are or how they fit into the big picture."

But Oscar could see that Nicholas was not fully convinced.

"Tell you what, tell you what… Let me work on this for a week and see what happens. I'll do it free of charge and if you don't see a big improvement by this time next week, I promise to scrap the thesis and write about something else."

He looked at Nicholas expectantly.

"Just one week, that's all I ask. I mean, things can't really get much worse, can they?"

Before he could response, Nicholas felt a timid tap on his shoulder. He had completely forgotten about Ana Tomi.

"Yes?" he said, exasperated.

"If you wouldn't mind, could you please introduce me to Axel? I'd like to find out what he does, exactly."

Too frustrated for words, Nicholas sighed dramatically, and set off down another long corridor, Ana hurrying along behind him.

"Wait right there till I get back," he shouted back at Oscar. "And don't touch anything."

# 34
# Downsizing demons

"Why do you keep all these?" Sally emerged from the hall closet with a bulging plastic bag.

"Ah, yes, my photos." Jake reached for the bag and peered inside, rummaging among the bundles, some tied with string, some bound with rubber bands.

"Do you keep every photo you've ever had?"

"Is that an accusation or a question?" Jake smiled at her, still sifting through the bag. "I like keeping a record of my life, actually," he said, not waiting for her response. "And I'd love to see more photos of you. I can't understand why you'd want to throw them all away."

"They're from the past, and they have no place in my life now. I needed to move on and let go of all that."

She looked at him again. "You know, it's healthy to let go of the past, Jake."

"Who says I haven't?" Jake was now down on the floor, pouring over a bunch of old photos from his teenage years. "Gosh, look at me there! What a hairdo."

Sally leaned over to look.

"Who's that with you?" she said, pointing to a petite fair-haired girl beside him.

"Oh, that's Cindy, my first girlfriend. We dated all through college. But then she moved away and married some accountant and had 2.5 kids. It wouldn't have lasted anyway. We were both far too needy and didn't really have any idea who we were."

He tossed the photo back into the bag and picked up another. He smiled.

"This one's of me and Jennifer in 1982. She was nice. A bit demanding, though. We lived in Ireland for a while and… Sal, what's wrong?"

Sally had gone quiet, and was sitting with her back to the wall, arms folded across her chest.

"This makes me uncomfortable," she said. "I can't help feeling that you're holding on to old stuff and can't let it go."

"Hey, maybe you're just jealous." He smiled at her. "Just because I haven't got rid of all my photos, doesn't mean that I haven't let go of my past, Sal—any more than you getting rid of your photos means that you've let go of yours."

"That may be true, but I still feel that it makes a difference, even if it's only a matter of cluttering up space with old things that you no longer use. If you went through these photos, I'm sure you could toss half of them and you'd probably let go of some old feelings, in the process. That can feel really good, once you've done it."

"Right, then. That's what I'll do." Jake gathered up the bag and the photos he'd tossed on the floor and headed down the hall to his office. "Perfect project for a rainy day. I'll be out in an hour or two, Sal."

He closed the door quietly and left Sally sitting in the hallway, half bemused and half annoyed that he had not put up more of a fight.

★ ★ ★

Cathy Compassion stood watching helplessly as two of her oldest and closest friends lugged their bags down the hill towards her.

"But why do you have to leave?" she said. "You've been here for ever. We're such a great team."

"Restructuring," said Casey Conditional forlornly. "If only I could make myself more indispensable maybe they'd keep me on, maybe they'd still find a use for me, or still like me. But I have no choice. I have to leave."

Cathy reached out to squeeze Casey's hand in sympathy.

"And Nige, what about you? What reason did they give for letting you go?"

Nigel Needful looked up from his suitcase, tears in his eyes. "They just said they didn't need me any more and that I was too much of a drain on the system. They said… they actually said I was *co-dependent*. Can you believe it? They said I needed to learn how to take care of myself in healthier ways, and that it would do me good to get out there to fend for myself."

He sniffed and wiped his eyes with the back of his sleeve.

"I don't know how I'm going to manage, I just don't. I don't know anyone out there to go to for help. I feel completely abandoned."

He turned to look beseechingly at Cathy.

"Cath, if you could just help me, I'd return the favour. You take care of me and I'll take care of you. Please? Could you? I don't want to leave."

Cathy was distraught.

"Oh, Nige, I'm so sorry. I wish I could, but I can't override a decision made by Command Central. They're always warning me about allowing my soft side to colour my judgement. They'd be on me like a shot if they found out that I'd helped you to stay. And then we'd both be tossed out." In dismay, Cathy turned to see two more of her friends coming towards her, one of them pushing a huge trunk in front of him.

"Vick, you're going too? I can't believe it. When did all this happen?"

"Oh, just in the past few hours, Cath," said Vick Timm. "Just like that, no warning. Some big clear-out, they said. How could they do this to me, after all I've done for them? I just don't get it."

"But how come you've got so much stuff?" Cathy pointed to the trunk.

"They said I had to take all my baggage with me, and I've been here the longest, so you can imagine... I don't know how they think I'm even going to get this lot onto the airbus. I can hardly push it, let alone lift it. These are the accumulations of a lifetime, you know. You can't just stuff em all into a rucksack and fling em over your shoulder."

"Well, couldn't you have left some stuff behind and got it sent on?"

"Nope. 'Parently not. All my baggage has to go with me. Even when I pleaded with them, and reminded them of all the hard times I'd had in the past. And all the times I helped out with emotional problems—like when that girl dumped His Lordship. Made no difference. They were utterly heartless. You know what? I feel used. I did so much for this place and now they're just going to discard me like a piece of old furniture."

"Same here." Ida No appeared suddenly behind Cathy, carrying two large hold-alls.

"Ida! Not you too? We have such great debates. Discussing the pros and cons of everything. Oh, this is terrible. Why do you have to go?"

"Not enough self-confidence in my work, they said. Always doubting my own decisions, second-guessing myself. The system's been revamped, you know, and the management is looking for different qualities in its employees these days. Young chaps coming in all cocky and confident. I dunno… I guess I just don't fit in any more."

She sighed heavily and sat down on her bags to wait for the airbus to arrive.

"Maybe I should have contested it. What do you think, Cathy? Should I have? Was I wrong to just leave without putting up a fight? But how could I have? I mean, I didn't stand a chance… Although I suppose I could have got a lawyer, or something. I still could, I suppose, couldn't I?"

Ida clasped her hands in an agony of indecision.

"No, you did the right thing, Ida. You'll feel much stronger for sticking with your decision to just leave. It's good to move on, you know. Make a fresh start."

She was interrupted by the approach of the Oxy Shuttle. With a whooshing sound, the big airbus moved slowly downstream and stopped beside the waiting group on the shore.

Cathy felt a lump in her throat as she watched her friends loading up their luggage. She was just reaching into her pocket for her pink lacy hanky when two more of her colleagues suddenly appeared beside her.

"We came to provide moral support," said Lee Nonmee, "so you wouldn't feel so lonely."

"Exactly," said Dee Cysiv. "Everything's going to be absolutely fine, Cath. We'll adjust. There's even talk of training for the rest of us, with a view to promotion."

"Oh?" Cathy was only half listening as the last of her friends boarded the airbus.

"Bye, Casey. Bye, Nige, Vick, Ida. Take care. You'll be missed." She stood waving as the door closed behind them and the Oxy Shuttle carried them slowly downstream and out of sight.

"What kind of training?" Cath turned back to Dee.

"Enhancement of our existing skills, new applications for them, healthier ways of interacting and communicating... all that stuff. Definitely a step forward for us all."

Lee put his arm around Cathy and they began walking slowly back up the hill.

"It's a whole new era, Cath. Very positive and upbeat. What's good for us is good for everyone—at least, that's what they're telling us. It will be strange without our old buddies for a while, but we'll support each other and adjust to the new program. Personally, I think it's going to be quite exciting."

# 35
# The appendix

"Right. This is the place. The only cul-de-sac in Highway 22. Like I said, a dead-end kinda guy. Well, I'll leave you here. You'll find him up ahead."

Nicholas strode off, leaving Ana standing, nonplussed, at the entrance to the cul-de-sac.

"Can I help you?"

Ana jumped. A small, wiry man had appeared out of nowhere behind her.

"Oh, you must be Axel. I'm Ana. I'm a student of anatomical studies and I was wondering if you could…"

"Course I can. Come this way, love. I don't have much work to do at the moment so I'll be glad to help you."

"Well, that makes a nice change," said Ana, with a sigh of relief. "How come everyone else around here is so unhelpful?"

"Oh, that's because they've got so many unresolved issues. The issues are in the tissues, you know. They just haven't figured that out yet. But don't worry about that lot. Come on down to my pad and I'll fill you in."

He led the way down the narrow street to a cosy chamber at the bottom of the cul-de-sac.

"What an interesting place," said Ana, looking around. "What exactly do you do?"

"Not much, according to that lot." He gestured back over his shoulder. "Because I'm pretty much off the beaten track, very few people take the trouble to find out what I do. So I'm glad you're here. Take a seat."

He pointed to a spongy protuberance along the side wall.

Ana sat down, her clipboard on her lap and her pen poised above the paper to take notes.

"Now, it's a bit complicated, but I'll try to keep it simple.

When I was a lad, my main job was to help rear white blood cells, called lymphocytes. Now, I'm more of a dispatcher, sending these cells off to other parts of the organism, when needed. We work together to fight off infections and help protect the system. We're a bit like a local Immune Inc., but we specialize in fighting off certain intruders associated with foods, drugs, microbes or viruses."

"But I've heard that sometimes your unit is axed in certain organisms because it gets all inflamed and causes problems. And people don't seem to think it's really needed at all."

"Well, again, that's because they're simply uninformed, I'm afraid. Here, follow me. I want to show you something."

Axel took off in the direction of the intersection, and then turned left. Ana hurried along behind him, barely keeping up as Axel beetled along. Within minutes, they arrived at what looked like a large entranceway, with soft doors that were in constant movement, making sucking sounds like a vacuum cleaner.

"This is a very important junction," said Axel. "It's what joins the Innercity Intestines and the main highway beyond— the junction between the Upper and Lower Colon Counties. It acts as a valve between the two, only allowing traffic through when it has been properly processed. It's manned by a guy called Leo Cecal, and he's very touchy. I'm glad to see he's not around at the moment. He and I don't get on too well." Axel looked around hesitantly. "Anyway, if there's too much stress or too many traffic jams, Leo gets cranky and he either allows too much traffic through at once, or he lets it build up to the point where everyone gets overly sensitive. And that's the problem."

"What do you mean?" Ana looked up from her frantic scribbling.

"See how close this place is to my unit?" Axel gestured back down the main thoroughfare to his cul-de-sac, which was clearly visible from where they were standing. "Well, when there's trouble here, my unit often gets blamed, and so we take the rap, instead of this guy getting it."

Axel grimaced in anger and headied back towards his unit.

"Pisses me off, that. And it happens all the time because this guy has such a nasty temper and the least little thing irritates him."

He turned to Ana as if she had challenged him on this.

"And even when there is a problem in my unit, it's usually because stuff backs up as a result of his lousy traffic control."

"But why don't you explain this to CC?" said Ana. "Surely this misconception should be corrected by them."

"It's pointless. I've tried. Leo just denies it and I end up looking foolish. He lives in denial, that guy. Needs to learn to let go more, stop hanging on to the past—old grievances, stuff like that."

They reached the cul-de-sac and Axel extended his hand to say goodbye.

"Thanks so much, Axel. This has been really helpful."

"Don't mention it. But when you're writing your thesis, just be sure to give me a chapter all to myself. I don't want to end up as an afterthought in the appendix. Ha. Good one, that, isn't it?"

And he was gone, leaving Ana wondering whether to laugh or not.

# 36
## Cold feet

The café was crowded when Sally arrived and it took her a moment to spot Cynthia in a booth at the back, waving at her through the bobbing heads. She pushed past the crowded tables, ordering a coffee from a passing waiter as she went.

"You look terrible," said Cynthia as Sally sat down opposite.

"Thanks. I feel terrible."

"What's up? You sounded very upset on the phone."

"I've, um, decided to leave Jake." Sally looked down at the table, unable to meet her friend's eyes.

"What? I thought things were going really well since you moved into his place. What happened?"

"Oh, there are just so many changes, Cynthia. He's not the same man any more. He's not the one for me. He's—"

"Hang on a second. Isn't that exactly what you wanted? I seem to remember you saying you wanted him to change."

"Yeah, but not like this. I never know what to expect from one day to the next. He's into all sorts of New Age stuff, and always exploring new things, and… it's very unsettling. He's changing so much and moving on and—"

"Ah, so that's it."

"What?" Sally looked up at her, barely noticing as the waiter arrived with her coffee.

"You're afraid he's going to leave you so you're going to leave him first. Classic."

"Of course I'm not." Sally blushed furiously. "That's ridiculous. I never said he was going to leave me."

"But that's what you're afraid of. Makes perfect sense to me."

"Cynthia, you don't know what you're—"

"Sal, shut up. You know how hard it is for you to be vulnerable with a man and to allow him to be powerful in his own right.

We've talked about this. It's hard for you to be with a partner who is your equal or, worse still, your intellectual superior. You love to take charge, fix things, find solutions—all things that men love doing, actually. Think about it... and stop shredding that napkin. It's not going to help."

"But he's *not* my intellectual superior," said Sally indignantly.

"Ha. See? Did you hear anything else I said? See how important that is to you?"

"But I—"

"You attracted a man who's actually a perfect match for you. Jake was easy-going and malleable to start with, and you were able to be in control of things and take charge of his health. But now that he's taking control of his own life and making healthy new choices of his own, you feel as if he no longer needs you and that you're being left behind. It's called co-dependence, you know—meeting each others' needs while ignoring your own stuff. You're feeling vulnerable and you don't like that feeling."

Sally glared defiantly at her, unable to speak.

"Sal, sweetheart, don't be afraid of getting closer. It's what this is all about. Jake loves you..."

Tears spilled out over Sally's cheeks and Cynthia reached over with her napkin to wipe them away.

"I knew you'd need that napkin. Look, it's okay. This is good. You need to soften, sweetheart. Otherwise you're never going to get the kind of love you really want, or the closeness and the incredible intimacy that come from being free to be yourself, just as Jake is learning to be. It's scary, I know, but it's the best. And he's everything you've always wanted."

"Yeah, but..." Sally was crying too hard to continue.

"Relationships are like relay races, you know. One partner gets ahead and then reaches back to pass the baton to the other, then it's the other way around. It's all about growing together, and that's what makes it exciting. Think how bored you'd be if things never changed or evolved? You'd be out of there, looking for a new challenge. It's what you've always done."

"When did you get to be so wise?" Sally looked at her, blowing her nose loudly.

"I've learnt the hard way, just like everyone else. And I know you. I know how you do this dance around intimacy, avoiding it at all costs because it's unfamiliar and because you don't think you deserve to be loved for who you are, rather than for what you have to offer."

"But I just don't know how to do it, Cynth. How do I move forward? And how can I be sure he's the man for me?"

"The one you're with is always the right one for what you need to learn at that time. He's there to show you what you most need to learn about yourself. As for moving forward, that's for you to work out in the moment, and in every moment, with Jake. You have to be willing to express your emotions all the time, telling him how you feel and telling him about your fears."

"But that will—"

"No, it won't. I know what you're going to say. Acknowledging your fears may be scary and make you feel horribly exposed, but it won't damage the relationship. Trying to keep them hidden is what will destroy it. Expressing your fears and allowing yourself to be vulnerable is the key to intimacy. There is nothing like it, Sal, for bringing two people closer together."

Cynthia reached across the table and squeezed Sally's hand.

"You've got to experience it. Trust me. It's the only way."

She signaled to a waiter.

"Let's get you a fresh cup of coffee and then we're going shopping for some sexy lingerie."

# 37
# De-programming denial

"Come in," said Brian, waving Jeremy into the CC office. "You know how busy we all are right now, so please make this brief." He gestures towards a seat, tapping his pen on his notepad as he waits for Jeremy to sit down.

"Well, um, it's about the organism's programming," says Jeremy, nervously shuffling his notes. "Lily showed me all the old negative stuff that's buried in the Top Secret files and she says it could potentially be accessed and changed into more positive programming, which would be good for everyone, right? And I'd like to work on that, if it's okay with you."

"That's very commendable, Jeremy, but how exactly do you plan on doing that? This is deeply engrained stuff, you know, and it's also highly sensitive material. It takes more than a little sifting through old files to figure out how things work and how to positively re-program the system with the necessary delicacy and awareness."

"Yes, I know, Sir, I know," says Jeremy earnestly, sitting forwards in his seat. "But I think I can do it, really I can, and it seems to me, with all due respect, that we don't have a lot to lose by my trying."

"Don't be so sure, son. There's a reason those files are Top Secret, you know. The programming can't be messed with and if it's not expertly handled things could get an awful lot worse than they are, believe me." He pauses, checking the bank of monitors behind him. "Tell me how you'd go about this, exactly."

"Okay, well, obviously I'd do all the necessary research first—find out what's in there and how it has affected the system physically and mentally. I'd catalogue all the data and identify the most significant recurring patterns produced by the programming. Then I'd focus on the emotional component and look at the breakdown of the various reactive patterns that developed in the early stages of the programming. I think that's the key, Sir." Jeremy sifts through his notes excitedly. "I'm beginning to understand how this conditioning can diminish self-worth and how that is the key to living a healthy, balanced life. We come to all kinds of negative conclusions about ourselves when our needs are not met or when someone treats us badly. And that distorts who we are, affecting the choices we make in life and causing us to avoid the very things that would bring us the most fulfillment. Then we—"

"Whoa, Jeremy." Brian holds up his hand. "I appreciate your enthusiasm, but let's keep this practical. What will you actually do to produce positive results? Have you developed some kind of software? And what kind of resources would we need to support the new programming?"

"Nothing! No, I mean, there's lots I can do but you wouldn't need any new resources. Look, I've got it all worked out..." Jeremy feverishly rifles his notes, extracting a large sheet of paper that he places on the desk in front of Brian.

"I've done a flow chart of the process." Jeremy points to a diagram of arrows and boxes. "I've worked out the sequence of things and the knock-on effect of the very early programming. See here, for example, how it goes from a particular incident in childhood to a feeling, to a decision about self-worth and then on to certain choices resulting from that? And you can see here, if you look at this other line, how His Lordship would have chosen a completely different career if his confidence hadn't been shaken by something that happened when he was 6. The programming was responsible for that. And we can change it, Sir! Different programming, different outcomes."

"Plan of action, Jeremy... specifics? I'm out of time, here." Brian looks pointedly at his watch.

"Just two more minutes, Sir, please. This is the best bit." Jeremy pauses for emphasis. "Based on my research, I believe that when we change the programming, we can change our circumstances—literally! We can get back in control of things.

All we need is the right software. And I've developed something that will activate the data buried in the Top Secret files and enable me to manipulate them. Practically speaking—" Jeremy raises his hand just as Brian is about to run out of patience—"this means that life will start to get easier and more rewarding for everyone, especially you."

"How much time would you need to run some trials with this software?"

"But I don't need t—"

"Jeremy, this is not up for debate. I want you to finish your research, catalogue the various programming components and then apply your new software to see what happens—in demo mode. I want none of this going live in the system until I give you the go-ahead. Do I make myself clear?"

"Yes, Sir." Jeremy looks glumly at his papers but then looks up brightly as an idea occurs to him. "Just one more thing, Sir."

Brian sighs. "What is it?"

"I've been leading meditation and leadership classes, as you may know, Sir, and they're having a profound effect. I've seen wonderful changes in everyone, with less stress, a more positive outlook, and greater awareness, mutual respect and acceptance."

"Sounds very lovey-dovey, Jeremy, but I'm not really interested in that stuff, you know. My focus is on the smooth, logical running of things, here."

"What I'm suggesting, Sir, will help with all that. If I can encode these same principles into the software, then the entire organism will operate more effectively. If I, um, were to run a little live test with this, Sir, surely that couldn't do any harm, could it?"

"Do the work, Jeremy, and bring me the software for testing, then we'll see. I'll give you clearance to the Top Secret database for one week, which should be plenty of time to put something together. Here's the access code." Brian reached for a piece of paper, wrote down a number and handed it to Jeremy. "Now, that's all I have time for. Please see yourself out."

★ ★ ★

Armed with his notes, Jeremy heads back to his work station, muttering to himself. "Why is there such resistance to change around here? You'd think everyone was addicted to pain and drama or something, the way they cling to old habits. I mean, it's not as if things are running smoothly the way they are. And why do we all have to be so careful, so afraid of making mistakes? It creates so much bickering and negativity." He smiled to himself. *Now who's being negative*, he thought.

Back at his desk, he puts down his notes and turns on his computer. "I'll show them. I'm not going to let a little resistance put me off. It's just a test of my conviction in myself and I know I can do this."

"Glad to hear it."

Jeremy looks up, startled. A young female stands in his doorway, dressed in pink leggings, short black skirt and a slinky multi-coloured top brimming over with voluptuous breasts. Her shiny dark hair is pulled into a spiky ponytail on top of her head. Her eyes are rimmed in bright green eye shadow, her eyelashes are an inch long, and her lips are encased in metallic blue lipstick.

"Who are you?"

"I'm your new assistant. Genna Gene. Brian sent me to help you with your research."

"Wow. That's amazing. And there I was thinking he was against the idea."

"Nah. He's just careful, is Brian. I mean, he's, like, responsible for everything, so he gets the rap if things go wrong. Which they do, lots." Genna flops down on the chair opposite Jeremy. "So, wanna get started? We've only got a week and there's a lot to do."

"Boy, for such an inefficient place, word sure gets around fast," says Jeremy. He motions for Genna to pull her chair up beside him, next to the monitor.

"So, what's your expertise? I mean, do you have any experience in software programming?"

"Yeah, kinda. My dad's Don Nathan Acid, also known as the DNA man. A real big shot. He's into genetic information and is pretty much responsible for the ee-vol-ootionary development of this place. God, I never hear the end of that friggin' evo-devo. I've learnt a thing or two from him about data storage an' stuff. But it's pretty boring, so I got him to use his pull to get me a summer job—just so I don't have to listen to him rant about his helixes, proteins and poly-thingamajigs."

"Oh, I get it. You're daddy's spoiled little brat and I'm supposed to keep you out of harm's way," says Jeremy, morosely. "Brian's not interested in helping me at all, is he? He's just doing a favour for your big-shot daddy, who I've never heard of, by the way."

"Oh, puh-*leeze*. Spare me the martyr act. Anyway, there's not much that can keep me out of harm's way. I love trouble, as the old man keeps telling me. He works behind the scenes, mostly, so I'm not surprised you haven't heard of him. Always has his nose buried in some scientific manual, if he's not chumming it with Ester Bonds, his oh-so-obnoxious assistant."

"What's wrong with her?"

"She wears these, like, loud, reeky perfumes that practically knock you over." Genna rolls her eyes dramatically and makes a gagging sound. "And the two of them are always in cahoots over some top-secret project. It's, like, sickening to watch. This will be much more fun, right? We can pull some strings and get this baby doing some wild new funky stuff."

"Sorry to disappoint you, but we can't do that. I have to create a prototype for Brian to verify before it goes live."

"Oh, sod that. We gotta run somethin' live, otherwise we'll never know if it works." Genna leans over the keyboard and starts typing manically. "All innovation involves risk. You can't be a pioneer and a wimp at the same time. Anyway, you said you knew you could do this, so what's the big deal?"

"Hang on a sec. What are you doing?" Jeremy leans forward, alarmed. "You can't get in there without the access code."

"Yup. Can, actually. You forget, my dad's high up, which means I know all the shortcuts. Now, let's see… If we open up the data relating to the first seven years, we'll get the gist of things." She continues typing furiously, with Jeremy looking flustered, a million questions in his head.

"First off," says Genna, "let's choose an area to work on—something key. What one thing could we change that would make a real difference in this place?"

"Uh, let me think." Jeremy looks perplexed, completely thrown by his sudden loss of authority.

"What one quality would really shake up this joint?" Genna prompts, fingers poised over the keys. "Think 'breakthrough', think 'personal empowerment'—all that good New Age stuff you spout in your leadership classes."

"Shit. Is this place bugged or what? How do you know all this stuff about me?"

Genna throws him a look of exaggerated boredom.

"Forget it. Let's stay focused here so I can think." Jeremy closes his eyes and rubs his temples. "Okay, I've got it. Fearlessness. Fear is what drives most of the decisions made in here and it throws everything off. Sam Stomach gets upset, traffic on Highway 22 gets all congested, Heather Heart throws a wobbly, Andrew Adrenal goes all hyper and the Kidney twins start whining. Everyone gets reactive and goes into survival mode, rather than thinking proactively about what's really best for the organism. If we could eliminate irrational fear from the programming, things would shift dramatically."

"Easy," says Genna, attacking the keys with a vengeance.

"Stop!" Jeremy pulls her hands from the keyboard. "Listen, this is my project, okay? I'm happy to have you help but this is not a game. You can't mess around in there without my permission. So let's be clear about that before we go any further."

"Gotcha, boss. You're the main man. So how would you like to address this fear issue?"

"Well, I'm working on some software but, um… why don't you tell me what you have in mind, then I'll decide on the best way to go." Jeremy sits straighter in his chair, gradually regaining his composure.

"Sublime," says Genna, turning to face him. "Fearlessness is, like, my favourite thing." She crosses her legs, jostling a lime-green flipflop up and down as she talks. Jeremy gets momentarily distracted by the sparkly gold nail varnish on her toenails and has to pull his attention back to the screen as Genna continues. "First, I go into the original programming, here," she points at a stream of data, "where fear first got imprinted. Then I do a search for all its derivatives, such as anxiety, self-doubt, lack of confidence, yada, yada, so we find all the different aspects of the organism that got infiltrated. We do a 'search and replace' with new programming to cancel out the old, and we use software to send mental stimuli via Command Central, prompting His Lordship to do the things he never dared to do when he had all that fear."

"We can't send anything via CC until we get approval," says Jeremy.

"No biggie. I'll use a multi-user dungeon and do a previsualization once I've rasterized the codecs. Simple."

"Uh, okay, but do a simulation first," says Jeremy. "I want to see what you come up with."

"Duh. That's what the multi-user dungeon *is*, boss—a simulation environment for software development. MUD, for short."

"Oh, right. Well, uh, what about cellular memory? Do we have enough capacity in the system for all this?"

"Oodles. I'll be uninstalling the old programs, which will free up even more room for the new stuff to be encoded. We'll need to defrag the whole system, too, but we can do that later."

"Will there be any side effects on the organism? I mean, will His Lordship feel any of this happening?"

"I friggin' well hope so. Not much point in it, otherwise. He'll feel a bit disoriented for a while but will probably start adjusting to it pretty fast. If you do your guru thing in your meditation class, that will help. I'd focus on the Heart Department, especially, if I were you. That's where most of the changes are gonna be felt, so you may find some resistance there."

"Any other suggestions, Genna?"

"Nope. That's it for now, boss. I'll get on with this, then, ya?"

"Okay, do it." Jeremy sighed. "I'll finalize this new software when you've finished playing around in the MUD."

# 38
# Going within

"Sam, I think you should go. It will do you good, bring down your blood pressure and relieve your stress a bit. Besides, you're the only one of the unit heads who hasn't participated." Sylvie stood facing her husband, brushing some fluff off his shoulder and looking at him with concern.

"It's just a load of New Age crap, Sylvie. Why on earth should I be bothered with that mumbo-jumbo? I've got more important things to do, such as running this place," said Sam, avoiding her gaze and looking seriously disgruntled.

"At least give it a try, would you, dear? You're far too obsessed with work and it's ruining your health. Plus you're turning into a boring old grouch. Trying something new would be good for you and would take your mind off things. Plus you're always bottling things up, which is very unhealthy. Remember what the others said about it really helping them relax and see things differently? Come on, I'll go with you." She held up her hand as Sam started to protest again. "Get over it. We're going. It's in the Pyloric Chamber, just around the corner. *Vámanos.*" Taking Sam by the arm, she marched him down the corridor towards the meeting room.

Soft music wafted towards them from the open door. Sam groaned and glared at Sylvie. "Hear that? New Age stuff. I told you."

Ignoring him, Sylvie stepped inside and looked around. The chamber was bathed in a soft orange light and about a dozen people were seated on cushions in a semi-circle on the floor. Sylvie nodded at those she knew—Lawrence Lung, Heather Heart, Andy Adrenal, Pete Pancreas and Oliver, Lily's assistant.

She sat down on a plump crimson cushion, crossing her legs and gesturing at Sam to sit beside her. Bristling all over and muttering to himself, Sam sat down, his legs stretched out awkwardly in front of him. "I can't do that cross-legged thing," he muttered. "Why can't they provide decent chairs?"

"You're starting to sound like an old man. Are you really so inflexible—in body as well as in mind? Could you just suspend judgement and condemnation until you've actually experienced something? At least Jeremy is trying to make things better around here. And—"

"Sylvie, I get the message. My bottom is numb already but I'm open to this being a blissful, mind-blowing, transformative experience, okay?"

"That's all I ask, dear. Ah, here's Jeremy now."

Wearing a long white cotton shift, Jeremy strides to the front of the room and takes his place on a large green silk cushion. He sits cross-legged and smiles warmly at the group.

"Welcome everyone, and a special welcome to Sam and Sylvie, who're joining us for the first time."

Sylvie smiles, nodding, and Sam grunts in response, looking at his feet.

"This is our sixth meeting and I've had great feedback from you all, so far. Anyone care to share what's happened for you since last week? What positive changes you've seen from doing this work?"

"Well, I've noticed a huge change," said Andrew. "I'm much better at handling conflict and no longer make unhealthy compromises. I'm not so hyper or depressed and am much more motivated about things in general. I've cut back on my hours and am finally able to switch off after work. I'm doing pretty well, all round, really."

"That's great, Andrew. Thanks for sharing that. What do you think brought about those changes for you?"

"Well, I'm beginning to understand how things work, Jeremy, thanks to your insights and what you said about the soul. We're much more in control of things than we think and we don't have to be victims. I realized that I've been living reactively most of the time, feeling out of control and blaming others, but now I understand that my circumstances are largely the result of my own negativity. So I'm learning to be more proactive and to make things happen the way I want them to, which is great fun, when you get the hang of it. And the techniques you taught us last week have really helped me to let go of blame and resentment, so I'm much more present."

"Wow. That's impressive, Andrew. Way to go, buddy." He looks around. "Anyone else?"

"Yes!" said Kyla. "Karl and I are feeling much more balanced and in synch. We've let go of a lot of toxic emotional stuff—you know, fears about what everyone thinks of us and how acceptable we are. And even though we're practically joined at the hip, we don't feel half as needy or co-dependent. Things just seem to be flowing an awful lot better."

"And the reason for these changes?"

"Well, like Andrew, we've been practising those techniques," says Karl, "exploring our fears and associated beliefs and then catching ourselves whenever we get reactive or disconnected from what we're feeling. Now, thanks to everyone else's efforts, there's far less toxic waste in the organism …and we've become much more efficient at processing it."

"Great work, you two. Working on ourselves benefits everyone in the organism, so the more of us that do that, the better." says Jeremy.

Sylvie shoots Sam a meaningful look.

"Before we move on to today's programme, perhaps you could tell us what you'd like to get from this session, Sam and Sylvie."

Sam stares fixedly at the floor as Sylvie clears her throat.

"I'm not exactly sure what you do here, Jeremy, but we were curious to find out, since we'd heard such good reports about your work."

"Well, let me start by asking you something, Sylvie: what would you most like to change in your life?"

"I'd like less stress and more down time—more peace of mind. Things have really improved, throughout the system, yet we still seem to be stuck in the old groove, feeling anxious and tense, even though there's no reason to be."

"Got it. Thanks, Sylvie. Sam? What would you most like to change? And please feel free to be frank. You're among friends here and we're all just trying to be the best that we can be and get more out of life."

"Yes, well…um." Sam's cheeks turn a deep shade of red and he fidgets with a shoelace.

Jeremy gets up from his cushion and hunkers down in front of Sam. He starts talking to him softly, barely loud enough for the others to hear. "I'm no guru, Sam, and I've had to learn humility the hard way. I've felt like the world's biggest loser all my life and yet I've been so full of arrogant pride that it's a miracle I didn't self-destruct. I'm still trying to figure out how things work, and you know what they say: you teach what you most need to learn. So here I am, as much a student as you, if not more so. So don't let your pride get in the way of you making a breakthrough, man. You've a lot to share and we'd be honoured if you were willing to do that. You play a crucial role in this organism, Sam, and we all respect and admire what you do. Now, though, maybe it's time for you to find more fulfillment in your life. What do you think, buddy?" Jeremy puts a hand on Sam's shoulder.

A full-body groan comes from somewhere deep inside Sam, who's bent almost double. Two huge teardrops fall onto his trousers and his shoulder start to shake.

Jeremy turns to the others. "Group hug, everyone," he whispers, beckoning them over.

"Nooooohhhwww." Sam vigorously shakes his head, unable to look at anyone as he swats the air to ward them off. But they gather around him anyway and envelope him in a massive bear hug. He starts to shake and tries to speak, his words punctuated by sobs.

"So much stress and t… tension… f…flak… no one un… understands… hold it all in… so mush fear… growing up… dunno how to be me…. Bloodyblubberingbaby… never li…li… live this down…"

"It takes huge guts to do this, man. Holding it all in is for cowards—those who can't face themselves or, worse, can't face who they dread to think they really are, underneath the façade. All our fears and doubts are just the result of our programming, Sam. They have nothing to do with who we really are. But they sure do get us all bent out of shape and tied up in knots. We're just trying to let go of all that, here—to fall apart, really, so we can put ourselves back together, our way. So thanks for being willing to unravel with us. There's no one more deserving of a breakthrough than you, Sam. And you play such a pivotal role that you affect everyone around you. That's a lot of power, man, and you can use it to really enhance your life and ours."

Sam nods, head still bent, and Jeremy waves everyone back to their cushions as he returns to his.

"Sylvie, could you dim those lights behind you, please? Thanks."

He turns back to the group. "In honour of Sam, we're going to do a special guided visualization on leadership, and I'm going to invite Sam to step in and lead it when he's ready—if that's okay with you, Sam."

Sam nods again.

"So, please lie down on your back, everyone, with your head on your cushion, and take some nice long deep breaths. Now, imagine yourself in a beautiful warm place, with clean air, everything functioning perfectly and everyone around you content, fulfilled, loving and passionate about what they do and who they are. No anger, no aggression, no resentments, just joyful willingness and dynamic cooperation. Imagine how you'd feel in that environment, with everyone trying to be the best that they could possibly be. How might you create that for yourself? How might you become the powerful entity you are meant to be?" Jeremy pauses to let everyone visualize this, then says, "Sam, would you like to take over?"

"I…I see that, I can feel it," he begins, falteringly. "And that sense of power… it comes from… my department. I only just realized that! That power, all that energy I've been feeling, I didn't know what it was. That's why I've put on weight—because I haven't known how to use it or what to use it for." He pauses in wonder. "The power is there for us all to use but we must find ways to harness it and use it positively, creatively, consciously. Otherwise it will just feed our fears and make us destructive." He pauses again, reflecting, then continues, his voice much stronger, this time. "Imagine that power being in every breath that you take. Feel it coming in…"

# 39
# Busting loose

It was hot and noisy in the pub, and it looked just as it had six months ago, the last time Jake had been here. The bar was lined with men drinking and watching a hockey game on a large-screen TV, their backs forming an almost impenetrable wall. Jake looked around for a familiar face, debating whether to fight his way up to the bar or take one of the few empty seats in the pews along the wall. He was just about to head for the latter when a heavy hand clasped his shoulder, startling him.

"Jake, ol' buddy, where've you been?"

Jake turned to find his old friend Charlie grinning back at him, pint of beer in hand. "Come and join me—over here."

Charlie led the way to a pew near the back, swaying a little on his feet and spilling some beer on the floor. He slid into the pew and immediately signaled to a passing waitress.

"The usual for you, Jake, my man?" Charlie asks.

"Yes, a beer, please... No, wait, I'll have a soda and lime."

"You can bring me that beer instead," Charlie says to the waitress, rolling his eyes at Jake. "*Soda and lime?*"

"I've kind of gone off the belly-building stuff since my cardiac arrest," said Jake, shrugging apologetically. *Damn*, he thought. *Why am I apologizing? I don't need to explain myself.*

"You've given up beer? I don't believe it. The man who used to practically drink me under the table... turned tee-totaler overnight?" Charlie looked at him in mock horror. "This can't be good for you, Jakey. What do you do for fun? We never see you in here these days. No more sports nights, no hockey games, nada."

"It was a coronary, Charlie, not just a hangover, you know. And it's changed my life, in ways that would be hard for anyone else to understand."

"Try me," said Charlie, draining his glass as the waitress returned with their drinks.

Jake smiled at the waitress and waited for her to leave before continuing. "My values have shifted, I suppose. Things that were important to me before just aren't important any more."

"Such as old friends, you mean?"

"No, Charlie, it's not like that. It's more to do with who I am inside. I'm living differently, doing things I enjoy rather than trying to be a hot shot, impress people or make scads of money. I'm connected to myself, in a way I never was before, and I feel much more fulfilled, more…" He paused, uncomfortable. "This is hard stuff to talk about."

"Jake, we've been buddies since high school. Credit me with a little more sophistication than a beer mat, okay?"

Jake grinned at him. "Oh, I dunno, Charlie, beer mats are excellent listeners, they're non-judgemental, you can lean on them and they never complain… That's more than most men have in their marriages—"

"Get on with the story."

"Okay. Well, you remember Sally, the woman I met last year?" Charlie nodded.

"She's completely transformed, Charlie. She started out doing the typical female thing—you know, trying to get me to eat right, lose weight, exercise and all that crap—and I just kept side-stepping it and acting as if it didn't bother me. But it really pissed me off. And I didn't like the way I handled it, either. Fact was, we weren't taking responsibility for our own lives. We were needy, trying to change each other in order to get our needs met, with the minimum upheaval. And we weren't looking at what was really going on inside. It was the same at work. I pushed myself to perform and do the manly conventional thing but my heart was never in it. I didn't realize how much it was all slowly killing me until I had the coronary. Best thing that ever happened to me, Charlie—not that I recommend it. I'm sure there are easier ways to get the message but I must have been particularly stubborn."

Charlie was listening intently. "And your relationship? What's it like now?"

"We're growing together, taking responsibility for our own stuff and taking risks, doing daring things, letting go of fears and insecurities. We're… authentic with each other, willing to be raw and exposed—to really be seen and loved. God, I know that sounds corny but I never realized how superficial and disconnected I was before. I was like a robot, going through the motions of living but never really, truly living. D'you know what I mean, Charlie?"

"Yeah, bud, I hear you. You've obviously got something special and I'm happy for you. You deserve it." Jake looked at his friend, touched by his sincerity.

"Thanks, pal. That means a lot." He cleared his throat and took a moment to study his soda. "You deserve it too. What's happening with you and Deirdre?"

"We split up, about four months ago. It wasn't working out. But…" He held up his hand. "I don't want to talk about it now, okay? Tell me more about you. What kind of work are you doing these days?"

Jake studied his friend's face, seeing a mixture of pain, confusion and loneliness in his eyes.

"Charlie, man, I'm sorry. I've been a lousy friend, so preoccupied with my own stuff."

Charlie shook his head. "We'll talk about me, bud, but not right now. Humour me, okay? It gives me hope to know that you've found what you really want—that it's possible to have all that good stuff in your life."

"I didn't believe it was possible either, before this. Listen, any time you want to talk..." They studied their beer mats intently for a few moments, then Jake cleared his throat before continuing.

"I've got my own personal coaching business now, which is great. I work with individuals and groups, helping them to live more authentic lives and to let go of the fears and beliefs that get in the way of their self-expression." He shakes his head in wonder. "God, I sound like a New Age commercial. But I'm still stunned by my life, you know. You'd think that loving life would be the most natural thing in the world and yet it took a near-death experience to shake me out of my self-destructive groove. We're even talking of starting a family in the next year or so. Can you imagine, Charlie? Me, the eternal commitment-dodger, thinking of becoming a dad?"

"When you had that heart attack, are you sure you didn't change places with some other normal guy out there in the ethers before you came back into your body?"

"You know, I've wondered the same thing myself," said Jake, laughing. "If so, I pity the poor bastard who got the old me back in his body."

Jake looked at his watch and pulled some notes from his wallet. "Charlie, I'm sorry but I gotta go. Drinks are on me." He stood up and leaned forward on the table. "Give me a call and we'll talk. Deal?"

"Yeah. Deal. Take care, buddy." Charlie did his best to look cheerful as Jake patted his friend's shoulder before turning to go.

As Jake walked towards the door, raucous cheers rose from around the bar as the hockey game progressed, voices competing to be heard above the general din. The smell of beer was making him feel sick, and the solitary drinkers, transparent in their attempts to numb their pain, were an uncomfortable reminder of the person he used to be. I don't belong here any more, he thought. And thank God for that.

Stepping outside, he felt his spirits lift as he breathed in the balmy evening air. Sally would be waiting for him at home and that was enough to bring the bounce back to his step. He decided to walk rather than taking a taxi, and he headed towards the park to take the scenic route.

The park was full of kids playing Frisbee, young mothers pushing strollers, and couples picnicking on the grass. Two boys, no more than 10 or 12 years old, were skate-boarding on the U-shaped ramp that Jake remembered using as a kid. He stopped to watch. They seemed to have endless energy, hurling themselves into the air, then twisting back onto the ramp with gravity-defying skill. He felt his blood stir with each pirouette, his body recalling the adrenaline buzz of being so fearlessly brazen. God, I used to do that, he marvelled. I must have had a death wish, even back then.

"Wanna try, Grandad?" One of the boys was calling out to him, skateboard extended in his direction. The other jeered from the ramp. "Yeah, Grandad, show us how it's done." They doubled over with laughter, gasping for breath.

He watched them, amused, and was about to turn away when he felt a spark ignite inside his brain, suddenly propelling his limbs towards the ramp. He felt overcome by a piercing sense of recklessness and his body seemed to have a mind of its own. His legs tingled and itched for movement, his heart quickened and he felt his face grow warm.

"Whoa, Grandad, you sure you can do this?" the younger one taunted him.

"Yeah, you got insurance?" the other one chimed in. But his grin froze as Jake reached for his skateboard.

"Okay, punks, stand back. I didn't want to embarrass you but you've asked for it." He waved them back to give himself plenty of space.

"Shit," muttered the older kid. "What if he, like, kills himself?"

A crowd seemed to have materialized out of nowhere, watching as Jake stepped onto the ramp. He took some deep breaths and visualized himself doing flips, smoothly, confidently, and landing squarely back on the board. He remembered the centrifugal force, the tug at his innards, the sensation of being suspended, frozen, in mid-air and then dipping back down, knees yielding, calves bulging, feet glued to the board.

The crowd did not exist. The park faded from his peripheral vision. His focus narrowed to the sloping wall of metal on either side. He started to move, rising higher and higher, momentum building inside and out. When he felt himself back in the zone, that place of utter oneness with the air, the elements, the shape of things, he launched himself, arching into the sky and corking back down, arms extended like a karate master as he rolled seamlessly up the other side. He flipped again and, in that moment of magical suspension, he felt a burst of exhilarated freedom deep in his gut. He let out a victory yell as he pivoted, and felt a huge ball of angst dissipate into the waiting air, leaving a spacey lightness in its place.

The crowd cheered and he felt himself slowly mesh back with his surroundings. He gradually coasted to a stop and jumped down from the ramp, scooting the skateboard back towards the boys.

"That was cool," said the younger one. "My dad would never do that."

*Neither would I …normally*, he thought. *What the hell came over me?*

He waved at the boys and set off towards home again, his legs like jelly. His centre of gravity felt different, too, as if he'd made some profound internal shift that affected his physical and emotional equilibrium. *What was going on?* Something had taken over his mind and body when he pulled that stunt. Ever since his heart attack, his body seemed to be doing unpredictable things, beyond his control. He couldn't help wondering who was really in charge.

★ ★ ★

Picking himself up off the floor, Jeremy looked dazed and dizzy.

"What the heck was that? It felt as if His Lordship was on a rollercoaster. Knocked me clean off my feet."

He looked at Genna, cool as a cucumber in front of the computer. It slowly dawned on him what had happened.

"Genna, I warned you about clearing stuff with me first. What have you done?" Jeremy scanned the monitor for the data commands Genna had just fed into the system.

"Calm down, boss. I just sent an impulse through CC to momentarily blow the fear circuits. And it generated a little fearless action, that's all. I encrypted it, though, so they won't know where it came from."

"That's it. You're fired. Out." Jeremy pointed towards the door.

"Did you hear about the party?" asked Genna, unfazed.

"What party?"

"Sam Stomach is having a party to celebrate."

"Celebrate what, Genna?"

"His newfound empowerment. Sylvie says he's a changed man. I wonder if our work here could have had anything to do with it…"

"He did that in the meditation group, actually."

"Ah, yes, but Sylvie just sent out an e-mail saying Sam had an amazing experience while His Lordship was doing somersaults— something to do with letting go of his life-long fear of rejection and finally being able to express himself from the heart. She said she's never seen him like this—warm, open, *fearless*, she said. Interesting, huh…?"

★ ★ ★

Jake felt buoyant and strong as he let himself in the front door. The wobbliness in his knees had gone and his whole body was tingling.

"Sal? I'm home!"

"Up here, darling," Sally called from upstairs. "In the bedroom."

*Good*, thought Jake. *Exactly where I want you.*

He took the stairs two at a time and burst through the bedroom door with a radiant smile.

Sally was on the bed, reading the newspaper.

"Wow," she said. "What have you been up to? You look… different."

Jake scooped the paper off the bed and threw it on the floor. He looked at Sally's smiling face, the rumpled bedcovers, the simple domesticity of their home, and he thought his heart would burst out of his chest with happiness.

"Sal…" he said, a world of words wanting to be expressed, but that was all he could manage. He took her in his arms and lowered himself onto the bed, kissing her neck, her shoulders.

"I'm so glad you're home, darling," she said, her hand on his chest. "Really home."

# 40
# Outward bound on the greatest journey

The vast Penile Centre was packed to capacity and the air crackled with anticipation. Stretching as far as the eye could see, millions of youngsters sat, transfixed, listening to the man addressing them from a stage at the front of the auditorium. Percy P stood tall and confident in front of a large microphone, looking rested and relaxed after his recent holiday. He scanned the rows of excited recruits, making eye contact with a few in the front rows.

"Okay, gang, this is it!" Percy's voice reverberated throughout the vast auditorium. "We've been told by Command Central that today is the day for our most important mission. It's what you've all been waiting for—the chance to make a meaningful difference. But, as you know, only one of you will succeed in this mission. Everyone else… well, what can I say. It's a bit like going to war. Not everyone makes it but I know you'll all make a heroic effort trying."

A buzz of excitement washed over the audience and several hands shot up simultaneously.

Percy waved them back down. "I know you have questions but obviously I won't be able to answer you all. I'll take four questions and then we'll have to prepare for mission launch." He scanned the rows again and pointed to a particularly eager blond-haired, blue-eyed youngster bouncing up and down with excitement. "Go ahead."

"What determines who makes it, Sir? Is it to do with our fitness level? Will it make a difference if we train harder beforehand?"

"Well, son, I'm not sure anyone can really answer that one. Provided you're all healthy, it's really a bit of a lottery. You're all strong swimmers so I'd say you've all got an equal shot at this."

"Next." Percy points at another eager beaver in the front row.

"Could you explain the launching process and what happens when we arrive at our destination?"

"Yes." Percy turns to a large projection screen behind him on the stage. "You will be launched into the receiving module, here..." He points to a diagram on the screen. "...at a speed of up to 200 inches per second. So remember to wear your helmets. Once inside, the race is on. Only about 100 of you will find the most strategic place for locating the target, which looks like this." He points to another diagram. "You'll have to fight your way up this canal and then go left or right—your choice—to find the target. The lucky winner must then infiltrate the target and fuse with it. And that is what I call a seminal moment."

"Next." Percy nods at someone in the second row.

"How long have we got?"

"You've got up to 24 hours, unless someone beats you to it. After that, you can all abort the mission as the target will no longer be receptive."

"Last question." Percy gestures to a freckled redhead in the fifth row.

"How do you know that today's the day?"

"There are certain key criteria that must be met for this particular mission to succeed, otherwise it's a complete waste of your time and effort—not to mention all the lives lost. The target is only receptive at certain times of the month, plus His Lordship needs to be in the right place, at the right time, for contact to be made. CC received an e-mail from Eyes&Ears this morning, saying that all the conditions were perfect, so it's a rare opportunity for you to make your mark."

Percy pauses, surveying the assembled masses. "Estimated time of departure is 8-10pm, so you've got five hours to prepare. Practise your breast stroke, crawl, wriggle or whatever you're best at, and take some time to sit quietly, reflecting on what you'll do if you end up being The One. This is a significant moment in history, small stuff, so give it your best shot. I'll be manning the launch from my station and I'll be rooting for you. Good luck!"

# 41
# Up close and personal

"Good book?"

"Yes, but not *that* good." Jake dropped his book on the floor and rolled over to face Sally as she got into bed beside him.

"What's it about?"

"Can't remember," said Jake, kissing her shoulders.

"But Jake, you only just put it down…"

"Yes, but then you got in and nothing else mattered. It's all a complete blur to me now."

"Silly man." She smiled at him and kissed the top of his head.

Then, suddenly serious, "Jake, I wanted to talk to you about something."

"Can't you see I'm busy?" He ran his fingers lightly over her neck, down her back and along her arm.

"Oh, gosh, that's… wow… oh, that's lovely…. It feels as if every nerve ending in my body is vibrating."

"As it should be," said Jake, continuing his feathery touch down her torso, along her left leg and down to her ankles.

"So, you wanted to talk?"

He brushed the soles of her feet with his fingertips.

"What? Ahhhh… Oh… no, it can wait… oh, don't stop. That's incredible… there's energy running up and down my legs, and I can feel amazing heat from your hands. What are you *doing*?"

"Just getting in touch."

Jake slowly drew his fingers over her stomach and up around her breasts, barely skimming the surface of her skin.

Sally moaned again, arching her back and sinking deeply into the pillow.

Jake ran his finger through her hair and whispered in her ear, "So, let's talk."

"What? Oh, um, yes. Well, I…"

Sally brushed her hair out of her eyes and turned to face him, her body still trembling from the massage. All of a sudden, she felt like crying. "Jake, I… I just wanted to tell you…"

"Yes, sweetheart. Tell me."

Jake stroked her face, his gaze steady and strong.

"I, um, wanted to tell you just, um, how much I love you, and how proud I am of what you've done, and…"

A wave of grief swept over her, choking off her words and leaving her gulping for air.

"It's okay, sweetheart. Tell me everything. Let it all come out."

"I just have so many, um, fears—fears that you'll grow beyond me and… and that you won't nee… need me any more, and that I'll have nu …nothing to give you and that as s…soon as I really open up my heart you'll leave."

She gulped convulsively, her stomach heaving with each spasm of grief.

"I'm sorry," she wailed. "I don't know why I'm so upset, I just…"

"Shhhhh, it's okay." Jake stroked her cheek, brushing away tears. "Just let it come. You've been holding it all in for far too long. Let it out, sweetheart. It's safe here."

A raw, ragged wail came from deep down inside her as Sally curled into a ball and Jake enfolded her in his arms. He rocked her slowly as she cried out her past, sweat running off her body as the energy of release coursed through her. Finally, she grew still, the last gulping sobs purging the remnants of grief as she relaxed into exhaustion.

"Oh, Jake, I…"

"Don't you dare apologize, Sal. I never want anything less than your whole heart—the love, the grief, the wounds, the fears and the doubts. Nothing less than that will do, now. Don't you see? Nearly dying showed me how to really live, and life is far too short for anything but the naked, raw truth. The only way we can truly grow together is to share our deepest thoughts and feelings, our niggling resentments—everything that might get in the way of our love. And out of that comes the deepest possible intimacy you can imagine. Like now."

He was inches from her face, staring intently into her red-rimmed eyes, her sweaty body crushed against his.

"Can you feel it?"

"Yes. Oh, God, yes. I can feel your heart. I can feel mine!"

She sat up, astonished at the realization.

"I've never felt my heart like that before. I can really feel it!"

Jake smiled at her lovingly. "And what does it feel like?"

"Like, I don't know... like a flexible, swelling, physical thing that can actually open and close. I never knew it could. I thought that was just an expression—you know, opening up your heart. But I can really feel it open. And there's so much in there."

She sank back down onto the pillow, a shadow of doubt crossing her face.

"I feel as if I could cry for a year. So much stuff from my past that I never knew was still in there. Old hurts, huge sadness, never getting enough love, always trying to make it not matter, being practical and sensible instead... I can feel it all. Jake, maybe I'm just too damaged for a healthy relationship. I think that's my biggest fear—that I won't ever be able to get beyond all this stuff from my past to have the kind of life and love that I want. I've spent so long keeping it all buried so that no one would find out who I really was, so that it wouldn't get in the way, but look where it got me. I feel flawed."

"You're not flawed, Sal. You're just hurt."

"But maybe I'm too hurt to ever really heal. Maybe—"

"Maybe you need to think less, feel more. And maybe you just need to open up to the possibility of being loved for who you are, no matter what that is. Do you think you could give that a try?"

She looked at him in wonderment.

"You really... you really love me, don't you?"

"Yes, I really do, Sal. And there is nothing you could do or say that would change the way I feel about who you are—here."

He placed his hand on her heart and drew her hand to his.

"This is all that matters, Sal. Forget about being right, forget about our conditioning, about what we should or shouldn't do. This is life right here, inside us, and nothing should get in the way of its honest expression—no matter how hard or scary that might feel sometimes. That, at least, is how I want to live. And that is the deepest, most meaningful commitment I could possibly make to you …in addition to marrying you, of course."

# 42
## Spermathon

"Mind if I watch?" Jeremy stood in the doorway of Percy P's office.

"Not at all. Come on in. You must be Jeremy. I've heard about you."

"I bet you have," said Jeremy, laughing. "Lily put me on one of your shifts when you were on holiday and I screwed up magnificently. She wanted to teach me a lesson in humility but it was more like an exercise in humiliation by the time Edgar Ego had finished with me. It would be good to see a real pro in action."

"Be my guest," said Percy, waving him to a seat. "You're just in time for the big event. You know Teddy, right?" He gestured behind him, where Teddy Testosterone was lounging in his chair, his fire stoked and ready to go.

"I certainly do. Hi, there, Teddy. How's it going?"

"Yo, Jeremy. Still causing trouble with the Ego-meister?"

"Nah, we're best of buddies now. He loves me."

"Yeah, right." Teddy snorted.

"We're approaching lift-off, as you can see from the dial here," said Percy, pointing at the Penis Panel. "And on this monitor here, you can see all the little sea-men getting ready for the launch." He pointed to a screen filled with a multitude of tiny helmeted bodies, jostling for space.

"Where are they all and how come I didn't see them when I was here?" said Jeremy.

"You must not have switched on this monitor. It shows what's happening inside the penile launch pad, which is where these guys are right now."

Percy starts working the levers, expertly switching from one to the other as the pressure mounts.

"Getting close now," he said, leaning into a microphone attached to the launch-pad monitor. "Small stuff, get ready. We have about 20 seconds to go."

The monitor seemed to come to life, with millions of little bods falling all over each other, desperate to get to the front line.

"Final countdown: 10, 9, 8…" Percy's hand vibrated from the pressure but held steady on the green lever. His other hand was poised on the red lever, ready to activate it.

"…5, 4, 3…"

Percy released the green lever, simultaneously engaging the red one.

"…2, 1, lift-off!"

He pressed a large red, arrow-shaped auto-eject button and the teeming masses on the monitor instantly became a fuzzy blur as they were catapulted from the penile launch pad.

"That's it. They're off."

"Wow. I certainly missed the show last time," said Jeremy.

"Well, usually that's all you see, and it gets a bit boring after a while, but this time is rather special. One of those little swimmers will engage with the target and a new organism will ultimately result. So it's a pretty significant mission."

"Can we see what happens next?"

"'Fraid not. Once they're launched, they're in foreign territory and we have no surveillance capacity over there. We'll have to wait for feedback from CC."

★ ★ ★

*It was dark, warm and hellishly slippery in the receiving module, and the tiny helmeted swimmers were frantically wiggling upstream. Several million had got knocked out upon impact, and numerous others were disoriented and dizzy, clinging to the walls and unable to get going at all. A core group of some five million were in the lead, swimming strongly up the channel towards a major V-junction. Half turned left, the other half right. Both routes curved around, each leading to a long, wide corridor that ended in a cul de sac. The group that had turned right continued valiantly down the right-hand channel, searching frantically for the target. Within seconds, they reached the end of the corridor, with no target in sight. They knew immediately that they were toast and they collapsed in collective defeat. The other group was speeding down the left-hand corridor, some falling by the wayside from exhaustion and others barely keeping up. But one core group still forged ahead, several thousand strong. Suddenly, at the end of the corridor, they saw the target—a round, egg-shaped form that pulsed slightly. With renewed vigour, the group wiggled urgently towards their goal, quickly surrounding the soft form and feverishly seeking entry. Only one would make it, they knew. And one did. Unable to believe his luck, a blond-haired, blue-eyed little fella found a tiny opening in the target and managed to wiggle inside. Instantly, the entry hole sealed over and he knew he was safe. He'd made it! He was The One.*

# 43
# Mission accomplished

"Wow. I think something happened there, don't you, Sal?" Jake collapsed onto his back in bed beside Sally.

"It most certainly did, my love, yes."

THE END

(or maybe just the beginning...)

# Glossary

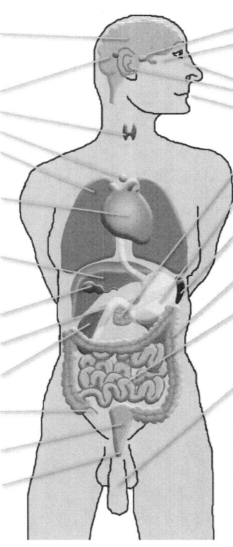

**Command Central**
*Brain*
Brian Brain
Crystal
Dr Medulla

*Pineal gland*

*Thyroid*

*Thymus*

*Lungs*
Lawrence Lung

**The Heartland**
*Heart*
Heather Heart
Arnie Aorta
Arthur Artery

*Liver*
Lily Liver
Oliver
Brendan Bile
Chloro Phyll

*Gallbladder*
Billy Gallbladder

*Adrenals*
Andrew Adrenal

*Kidneys*
Karl and Kyla Kidney

*Appendix*
Axel Appendix

**Rectum Region**
*Rectum*

**Anus Alley**
*Anus*

*Hypothalamus*

*Pituitary*

**Eyes 'n' Ears**
*Eyes*
*Ears*

*Mouth*
Pontius Palate
Taste Buddies

*Pancreas*
Pete Pancreas

*Stomach*
Burnie, George Gastric
Sam & Sylvie Stomach

*Spleen*
Sophie Spleen

**Colon County**
*Large Intestine*

**Highway 22**
*Small Intestine*
Ace Acidophilus
Barney Bifidus
Candice Candida
Frederick Fungus

*Penis*
Percy P.
Teddy Testosterone

*DNA*
Jeremy Gene
Genna Gene

*Mind*
Edgar Ego
Millie Me

*Lymphatic System*
Nicholas Nodes
Larry Lymphocyte

OLGA SHEEAN

**ACIDOPHILUS** *Ace Acidophilus*

Lactobacillus acidophilus is one of several probiotics (friendly flora) that populate the gut and promote immunity and proper nutrition in the body. These friendly flora also aid digestion, produce natural antibiotics, manufacture vital nutrients and regulate elimination. Acidophilus, together with Lactobacillus bulgaricus, Lactobacillus bifidus and other friendly bacteria, also balances digestion and is often used to treat diarrhea and constipation. If there are too few of these friendly bacteria in the gut, digestion can be impaired, reducing the nutrient uptake from our foods and weakening the immune system.

**ADRENALS**

*Andrew Adrenal*

The adrenal glands are tiny organs that rest on top of each kidney. They produce hormones (chemical messengers that regulate body functions) that have an impact on development and growth, affect our ability to deal with stress, and help regulate kidney function. The adrenals produce the hormones adrenaline and noradrenaline (also known as epinephrine and norepinephrine), which regulate the 'fight or flight' response in the body (the body's reaction to stressful events), as well as several other hormones that affect blood pressure and blood sugar levels, growth and some sexual characteristics.

At the psycho-emotional level, the adrenals are to do with being able to handle conflict—standing our ground when we are faced with other people's expectations, demands or pressures. When the adrenals are stressed, it usually means that we are making compromises or choices that don't really work for us.

**APPENDIX**

*Axel Appendix*

The appendix is a small pouch—like a tiny cul de sac—located at the point where the small and large intestines join. Formerly thought to serve no useful purpose, it is now seen as a tough soldier against infection, especially in those who have been exposed to certain types of radiation. Inside the appendix is lymphoid tissue, which helps produce the white blood cells that fight disease.

187

At the psycho-emotional level, the appendix is to do with back-up protection—the last resort if things get really out of hand. If the appendix gets inflamed or blocked, it usually indicates some kind of emotional overwhelm.

## BONES

*Mandy Bone Marrow*

The body's 206 bones provide support for the body, giving it shape, form and the ability to move and take action. They protect vital organs and, being attached to muscles, serve as levers to make movement possible. Bones are storage reservoirs for minerals and vitamins, and bone marrow is responsible for the production of new blood cells. Bones are living, changing structures that need calcium and weight-bearing exercise to build and maintain their density and strength.

At the psycho-emotional level, the skeletal system represents a way out, since it enables us to physically remove ourselves from painful, uncomfortable or unsafe situations. If we have problems with our bones, it can mean that we are not taking the appropriate action, or making the right moves, to keep ourselves safe and in the best possible place.

## BRAIN

*Brian Brain, Crystal, Dr Medulla*

The brain is the control centre for movement, sleep, hunger, thirst, sexual desires, mood, data analysis and virtually every other vital activity necessary to survival. It controls all mental functions, remembers past experiences and is the source of thought, moods and emotions.

At the psycho-emotional level, the brain is about simplifying complications and reducing things down to their essence. If we have problems with brain function, it usually indicates that things have become overly complicated, resulting in mental/electrical overwhelm.

## CANDIDA

*Candice Candida*

Candida albicans is a yeast that occurs naturally in the body but can quickly proliferate and take over all the healthy microorganisms, as a result of too many refined/sugary foods, the use of antibiotics, and stress. Numerous symptoms and chronic ill health can result. Normally found in the intestines, mouth, throat and genitals, Candida can burrow through the intestinal walls, enter the blood stream (where it emits numerous toxins) and reach any organ of the body, causing numerous symptoms and problems, such as abdominal gas, headaches, extreme fatigue, cravings for alcohol and sweet things, anxiety, vaginitis, rectal itching, brain fog and difficulty concentrating, hyperactivity, mood swings, diarrhea, constipation, acne, depression, sinus inflammation, PMS, dizziness, poor memory, earaches, low sex drive, muscle weakness, irritability, learning difficulties, sensitivity to fragrances and/or other chemicals, cognitive impairment, thrush, athlete's foot, sore throat, indigestion, acid reflux and chronic pain.

## CARBOHYDRATES

The two main forms of carbohydrates are sugars, also known as simple carbohydrates (such as fructose, glucose, and lactose), and starches, also known as complex carbohydrates, which are found in foods such as starchy vegetables, grains, rice, breads and cereals. The body converts most carbohydrates into the sugar glucose, which is absorbed into the bloodstream. As the glucose level rises in the body, the pancreas releases a hormone called insulin. Insulin is needed to move sugar from the blood into the cells, where it can be used as a source of energy. Complex carbohydrates are considered to be more beneficial for the body than simple carbohydrates as they provide more nutrients and are broken down more slowly in the body, resulting in more sustained energy production.

## CENTRAL NERVOUS SYSTEM

If the brain is like a central computer that controls all bodily functions, the nervous system is like a network that relays messages back and forth from the brain to different parts of the body, regulating the body's responses to internal and external stimuli. It does this via the spinal cord, which runs from the brain down through the back and contains threadlike nerves that branch out to every organ and body part.

At the psycho-emotional level, the central nervous system is like our personal radar system, keeping us alert to, and aware of, what's going on around us, in order to keep us safe. If we have problems with our central nervous system, it can mean that we are over-stimulated or that fears and insecurities have made us overly reactive or sensitive to our environment.

## DIGESTIVE ENZYMES

*Peggy Protease, Anton Amylase, Lyle Lipase, Larry Lactase, Celine Cellulase, Polly Peptides*

If the body cannot efficiently digest or process food, as can be the case for the elderly, or in times of stress or illness, it can be beneficial to take digestive enzyme supplements. The main digestive enzymes used to boost digestion and nutrient absorption are amylase (for digesting carbohydrates), lipase (for digesting fats), protease (for digesting proteins), cellulase (for digesting cellulose, the cellular tissue of plants) and pepsin (which converts proteins into smaller units called peptides). Lactase digests lactose (milk sugar). If we are unable to digest lactose, due to a lactase deficiency, we can become lactose-intolerant (unable to digest dairy products). If there is insufficient stomach acid, it can also be beneficial to take supplements of hydrochloric acid, which breaks down proteins, kills off potentially harmful bacteria/parasites in our food, controls yeast levels, and facilitates the absorption of minerals such as calcium and iron.

## DNA

*Don Nathan Acid*

Deoxyribonucleic acid (DNA) is a nucleic acid that contains the genetic instructions used in the development and functioning of all known living organisms and some viruses. The main role of DNA molecules is the long-term storage of information. DNA is often compared to a set of blueprints, a recipe or a code, since it contains the instructions needed to construct other components of cells, such as proteins and RNA molecules. The DNA segments that carry this genetic information are called genes (see GENES).

## EARS

The ear converts sound that enters the ear canal—from mechanical vibrations into electrical signals that the brain interprets. The ear also contains a fluid that is vital for balance.

At the psycho-emotional level, the ears are about hearing the whole truth and being able to handle it. If we have trouble with our hearing, it can sometimes indicate a need to block out certain issues or people that we feel we can't handle.

## EGO

*Edgar Ego, Millie Me*

According to Freud, the ego's job is to meet the needs of the primitive self (which wants whatever feels good, regardless of the situation), while taking into consideration the reality of the situation. The superego, on the other hand, is the moral/ethical part of us that's defined by our upbringing. The superego is often considered to be the conscience as it determines our sense of right and wrong. The ego can also be seen as the sum of all our beliefs: I am kind, selfish, fat, pretty, ugly; life is cruel, a struggle; people are loving, pretentious, jealous; I should be compassionate and loving; I should be tough and strong; I should show my emotions; I should hide my anger. This collection of fixed beliefs is what makes the ego and defines 'me', differentiating 'me' from others. Because we so closely identify with these beliefs, we tend to protect, defend and fight for them, even if they don't serve us in positive ways. We believe they make us who we are and anyone who challenges or judges them becomes our enemy. Dropping the ego therefore means dropping the limiting beliefs that obstruct our vision of vaster possibilities. It means opening our mind to the point where we can see that we are all one, despite our apparent differences.

## ENDOCRINE SYSTEM

The endocrine system is a collection of glands (adrenals, sexual organs, thyroid, pancreas, thymus, hypothalamus, pituitary and pineal) that secrete chemical messages called hormones. The hormones pass through the blood to the target organ, resulting in a chemical change in the body.

At the psycho-emotional level, the endocrine system represents the body's trauma centre. If physical, emotional, sexual or psychological trauma occurs, it will create a powerful electrical charge in the endocrine system, which can, in turn, 'blow our circuits'.

## EYES

The eyes work like a camera. Light passes through the lens of the eye and is 'recorded' on the back of the eye—the retina. The eye sends the picture to the brain, which then turns the picture the right way up and tells you what you are looking at.

At the psycho-emotional level, eyesight is to do with how we see or perceive life. Problems with our vision usually indicate an inability to see (or a resistance to seeing) things as they really are. Short-sightedness can indicate a difficulty in seeing the 'big picture', whereas long-sightedness can indicate a difficulty in focusing on the small stuff.

## FATS

The body uses fat as a source of fuel and energy, and fat is the body's main form of energy storage. Fat has many other important functions in the body, and a moderate amount is needed in the diet for good health. Fats in food come in several forms, including saturated, monounsaturated and polyunsaturated. Too much fat or too much of the wrong type of fat can be unhealthy. Fat makes up part of our brains, protects some of our joints and provides reserves for when we're sick. It is also needed for the absorption of fat-soluble vitamins A, D, E and K, and to prevent deficiencies of these vitamins. Fat also provides back-up energy if blood sugar supplies run out (after 4-6 hours without food), provides insulation under the skin from the cold and the heat, protects organs and bones from shock and provides support for organs, surrounds and insulates nerve fibers to help transmit nerve impulses, forms part of every cell membrane in the body, helps transport nutrients and metabolites across cell membranes, and makes building blocks needed for everything from hormones to immune function.

## GALLBLADDER

*Billy Gallbladder*

The gall bladder is a small, pear-shaped muscular sac, located under the right lobe of the liver. Here, bile secreted by the liver is stored until needed by the body for digestion.

At the psycho-emotional level, the gall bladder is to do with being decisive and having the courage to do what we know we need to do. If we have gall bladder problems, it usually indicates that we haven't managed to summon up the guts to take decisive action, for our own benefit.

## GENES

*Jeremy Gene*

Genes are the basic units of heredity and they hold the information for building and maintaining cells and passing genetic traits on to offspring. There are many genes corresponding to many different biological traits, some of which are immediately visible, such as eye colour or number of limbs, and some of which are not, such as blood type or increased risk of specific diseases. In cells, a gene is a portion of DNA (see DNA) that contains both 'coding' sequences, which determine what the gene does, and 'non-coding' sequences, which determine when the gene is active. When a gene is active or expressed, the coding and non-coding sequences are copied in a process called transcription. The molecules resulting from gene expression are known as gene products, which are responsible for the development and functioning of all living things. The physical development of organisms is basically the result of genes interacting with each other and with the environment.

At the psycho-emotional level, genes represent our psychological and emotional programming—how we have been programmed to think about the world and about ourselves. This programming, which is made up of beliefs, fears and perceptions handed down from generation to generation, determines how we see the world and what we think is possible for us in life.

## HEART

*Heather Heart, Arnie Aorta, Arthur Artery*

The heart is a chambered muscular organ that pumps blood received from the veins into the arteries, thereby maintaining the flow of blood through the entire circulatory system to supply oxygen to the body.

At the psycho-emotional level, the heart is to do with forgiveness and letting go of past hurts or grievances so that we can be at peace with ourselves. Heart problems usually indicate an inability to be emotionally flexible so that forgiveness of self and others can take place.

## HYPOTHALAMUS

Often called 'the brain of the brain', the hypothalamus maintains the body's status quo, regulating factors such as blood pressure, body temperature, fluid and electrolyte balance, and body weight. It organizes and controls many complex emotions, feelings and moods, as well as all motivational states including hunger, appetite and food intake, and everything to do with pleasure, including satisfaction, comfort and creative activities. It also produces neurotransmitters that relay information and instruction to all parts of the brain and body, directly influencing the pituitary gland. The hypothalamus is involved in the integration of physiological stimulation via all five senses—taste, smell, sight, sound and touch—which it then translates, distills and assembles into one discernible 'package', relating all the associated stimulation into one clear harmonious concept, memory and experience, thereby yielding a succinct, emotionally satisfying understanding and assessment of the experience itself.

At the psycho-emotional level, the hypothalamus is designed to enable us to make clear sensory evaluations so that we can communicate and manifest what we want in life.

## ILEO-CECAL VALVE

*Leo Cecal*

The ileo-cecal valve is a small muscle located between the small and large intestine, in the lower, right-hand side of the abdomen. This one-way valve allows our food to pass into the large intestine for further processing. The valve is designed to open and close, as required, but when it gets stuck in the open position, it causes a backwash from the large intestine into the small intestine, allowing fecal matter to seep into the blood. This creates problems as the small intestine is where the process of creating the blood/fuel to feed the body begins. When the valve gets stuck in the closed position, the process of eliminating waste is hindered. Both of these conditions create a toxic build-up that can cause problems in the body. A faulty ileo-cecal value is usually the result of stress and/or of eating the wrong foods, which can seriously affect the performance of the whole body.

At the psycho-emotional level, the ileo-cecal valve reflects an inability to properly digest information received (when the value is stuck in the open position), and an inability to let go/over-attachment to certain things, situations or people (when the valve is stuck in the closed position).

## INTESTINES/HIGHWAY 22

*Barney Bifidus, Frederick Fungus*

The intestines are the portion of the digestive tract between the stomach and the anus, and they are divided into the small intestine and the large intestine. The small intestine is about 22 feet long and this is where most digestion occurs and where most nutrients are absorbed. The large intestine is responsible for absorption of water and excretion of solid waste material. Food and waste material are moved along the length of the intestine by rhythmic contractions of intestinal muscles, called peristalsis. Waste is solid because most of the water has been removed by the intestines as it travels through them.

At the psycho-emotional level, the intestines are to do with making the distinction between what is healthy and what is toxic in our lives, and processing things accordingly. If we have problems in our intestines, it usually means that we have difficulty processing life, letting go of the past, and knowing what's best for us.

## JAWS

The jaws enable us to ingest and chew food in preparation for digestion. Without the movement of our jaws, we would have great difficulty nourishing or expressing ourselves.

At the psycho-emotional level, the jaws represent our ability to articulate what we feel and want. If we have tension in the jaws, it usually means that we have censored or bitten back our words, or avoided expressing what we feel to someone.

## KIDNEYS

*Karl and Kyla Kidney*

The kidneys are two small organs located near the spine at the small of the back. Their main purpose is to separate urea, mineral salts, toxins and other waste products from the blood. The kidneys also maintain the proper balance of water, salts and electrolytes, and filter the blood of metabolic wastes, which are then excreted as urine.

At the psycho-emotional level, the kidneys are to do with processing fears and toxic emotions so that the body is kept emotionally 'clean'. If we have kidney problems, it often means that we are holding onto our fears or we have trouble resolving conflicting emotions.

## LIPOTROPIC FACTORS

Lipotropic factors are substances that prevent excessive build-up of fat in the liver, hastening removal or decreasing any deposits that may have been made. These substances also increase the liver's production of lecithin, which keeps cholesterol more soluble, detoxifies the liver, and increases resistance to disease by helping the thymus gland to carry out its functions. Lipotropic factors include the B vitamins choline and inositol, an essential amino acid (protein) called methionine, and betaine hydrochloride, which increases stomach acid. Without lipotropics, fats and bile can become trapped in the liver, causing severe problems, such as cirrhosis, and blocking fat metabolism.

## LIVER

*Lily Liver, Oliver, Brendan Bile, Chloro Phyll*

The liver is the largest glandular organ of the body and it has numerous functions, including: the production of substances that break down fats; the conversion of glucose to glycogen; the production of urea (the main substance of urine); the manufacture of certain amino acids (the building blocks of proteins); filtration of harmful substances (such as alcohol or drugs) from the blood; storage of vitamins and minerals (vitamins A, D, K and B12); and maintenance of proper levels of glucose in the blood. The liver is also responsible for producing cholesterol, producing about 80% of the cholesterol in the body.

At the psycho-emotional level, the liver is to do with efficiently planning or orchestrating our lives so that they work for us and bring us benefits in accordance with the efforts we've made. It also relates to sudden insights and spontaneous solutions, as well as being a source of rage, frustration and anger when it is out of balance. If we have liver problems, it often means that we have difficulty balancing life's priorities or that we are doing too much for others, to our detriment.

## LUNGS

*Lawrence Lung*

The lungs remove carbon dioxide from the blood and provide it with oxygen. Every day, we take about 23,000 breaths, inhaling gases (including oxygen) that our cells need in order to function. With each breath, our lungs add fresh oxygen to our blood, which then carries it to our cells. The lungs also affect the pH (the degree of acidity/alkalinity) of our blood, filter out small blood clots formed in veins, and filter out gas micro-bubbles occurring in the venous blood stream, such as those created after SCUBA diving.

At the psycho-emotional level, the lungs are to do with being emotionally present. Every breath we take is designed to bring us back to neutral—to the present moment—a bit like the 'refresh' button on a computer. If we have lung problems, it usually means that we are emotionally blocked or in denial about some issue in our lives.

## LYMPHATIC SYSTEM

*Nicholas Nodes, Larry Lymphocyte*

The lymphatic system consists of organs (bone marrow, lymph nodes, spleen and thymus), ducts and nodes. It transports a clear, watery fluid called lymph, which distributes immune cells and other factors throughout the body. It also interacts with the blood circulatory system to drain fluid from cells and tissues. The lymphatic system contains immune cells called lymphocytes, which protect against antigens (viruses, bacteria, etc.) that invade the body. Besides providing a home for lymphocytes (B-cells and T-cells), the ducts of the lymphatic system provide transportation for proteins, fats and other substances via the lymph.

At the psycho-emotional level, the lymphatic system is to do with self-identity and knowing who we are. Problems with our lymphatic system can indicate a weak sense of self and difficulties being decisive about what we want/where we should go in life.

## MINERALS

Whereas vitamins are organic substances (made by plants or animals), minerals are inorganic elements that come from the soil and water and are absorbed by plants or eaten by animals. They are needed for the proper composition of body fluids, the formation of blood and bone, and the maintenance of healthy nerve function. Your body needs larger amounts of some minerals, such as calcium, which is required to build strong bones and teeth. Other important minerals include chlorine (which maintains body fluids, electrolyte balance and digestive juices), magnesium (which is needed for every major biological process, the use of glucose in the body, the synthesis of nucleic acids and protein, and for cellular energy), potassium (which works with sodium to control the body's electrolyte balance, promotes a healthy nervous system, helps maintain stable blood pressure and transmits electro-chemical impulses), and sodium (which, with potassium, helps maintain electrolyte balance and pH). Other minerals, such as chromium, copper, iodine, iron, selenium and zinc, are called trace minerals because only very small amounts are needed daily.

## PALATE

*Pontius Palate*

The palate is the roof of the mouth and it is made up of the soft palate, at the back of the throat, which prevents food from entering the nasal cavity during chewing and swallowing, and the hard palate, directly above the tongue, which helps form speech sounds and allows food to be chewed while breathing continues. Although the palate is not the fully responsible for the sense of taste (the tongue has most of the taste buds), there are some taste buds on the soft palate that contribute to the body's ability to identify the various flavours of foods. (See TASTE BUDS.)

At the psycho-emotional level, the palate is to do with healthy discernment and an appreciation for the good things in life.


## PANCREAS

*Pete Pancreas*

The pancreas is a gland that secretes digestive enzymes and hormones. It contains enzyme-producing cells that secrete two hormones—insulin and glucagon—which are secreted directly into the bloodstream and, together, regulate the level of glucose in the blood. Insulin lowers the blood sugar level and increases the amount of glucagon (stored carbohydrate) in the liver. Glucagon slowly increases the blood sugar level if it falls too low. If the insulin-secreting cells do not work properly, diabetes occurs. The pancreas produces the body's most important enzymes, designed to digest foods and break down starches. The pancreas also helps neutralize chyme (see STOMACH) and helps break down proteins, fats and starch.

At the psycho-emotional level, the pancreas relates to knowing our feelings and emotions. If we have problems with the pancreas (such as low blood sugar or diabetes), it usually means that we have difficulty getting in touch with our emotions or knowing what we feel about particular situations or people.

## PINEAL

The pineal is a small endocrine gland in the centre of the brain, directly behind the eyes. It produces the hormone melatonin, which regulates patterns of sleep and wakefulness. The gland is activated by light and it controls the various biorhythms of the body. It works in harmony with the hypothalamus gland, which directs the body's thirst, hunger, sexual desire and the biological clock that determines our aging process. The pineal may also play a significant role in sexual maturation, seasonal affective disorder (SAD) and depression.

At the emotional/spiritual level, the pineal gland, often referred to as the 'third eye', is associated with mystical powers and psychic abilities.

## PITUITARY

The pituitary gland is sometimes called the 'master' gland of the endocrine system, because it produces hormones that control the functions of the other endocrine glands. The size of a pea, it is located at the base of the brain and is attached to the hypothalamus by nerve fibers. The hypothalamus acts as the collecting center for information concerning the internal well-being of the body and it uses much of this information to regulate the secretion of the hormones produced by the pituitary.

At the psycho-emotional level, the pituitary is thought to relate to the mastery of our destiny and the achievement of our goals in life.

## PROTEIN

Protein is the body's builder, essential for growth, repair and the regeneration of cells. Healthy skin, hair, nails and internal organs depend on the right amount and form of protein in our diet. Protein is also required for muscle tissue, the transportation of nutrients and oxygen to our cells, and the production of antibodies. Protein is made up of 22 amino acids (the body's building blocks), eight of which can only be obtained from our food. Sources of animal protein include meat, fish, chicken, cheese, eggs and milk, whereas plant protein sources include soy, spirulina and hempseeds (which may reduce the risk of strokes, heart attacks and heart disease). Eating plant-based proteins may help prevent the build-up of arterial plaque, which can cause artery hardening and blockages. Due to the high levels of saturated fats and additives found in red meat, a plant protein diet is often considered to be a healthy alternative. However, depending on the blood type and constitution of the individual, different forms of protein may be required for different people.

## REPRODUCTIVE ORGANS/PENILE PANEL

*Percy P, Teddy Testosterone*

The primary purpose of the reproductive organs is to produce offspring. The female reproductive organs (mainly the ovaries, uterus and vagina) are designed to receive sperm from the male and provide a favourable environment for the development of a fetus, whereas the male organs (primarily the penis, testes and prostate gland) are designed to eject sperm into the female so that it can be fertilized by the female egg, resulting in conception. Both sets of organs are also designed to give pleasure (which, some would claim, is just another way to ensure that the species continues to reproduce).

At the psycho-emotional level, the reproductive organs are to do with creativity, passions and manifesting what we want in life. If this part of the body is dormant or blocked, we may have difficulty connecting with our passions or making our lives work. When it is active and healthy, it enables us to attract the people/things that feed our passions and creativity, thereby enhancing our fulfillment.

## SKIN

The skin is the outer covering of the body and it is the largest organ, made up of multiple layers of tissues. It guards the underlying muscles, bones, ligaments and internal organs. Because it interfaces with the environment, skin plays a key role in protecting the body from pathogens and excessive water loss. Its other functions are insulation, temperature regulation, sensation, synthesis of vitamin D, and the protection of vitamin B folates.

At the psycho-emotional level, the skin is about boundaries—knowing where to draw the line with others so that we make wise, healthy choices in our lives. If we have skin problems, it often indicates that we have difficulty creating or maintaining healthy boundaries or we have issues relating to our self-image, since our skin defines our shape and appearance to the world.

## SOUL

In many religions and philosophies, the soul is considered to be the spiritual or immaterial part of a living being, often regarded as eternal and believed to live on after death. It is usually thought to consist of one's consciousness and personality, and can be synonymous with spirit, mind or self. The soul is also considered to be the aspect of the body that gives it vitality. It is the life force of the body, the charging agent that gives animation and growth to the body. Some say that the body is the vessel in which this true form of life can manifest itself and that it is merely an abode for the soul.

At the psycho-spiritual/emotional level, the soul represents the higher, intuitive, wiser part of us that sees beyond the tangible reality of our physical world. If we are disconnected from our spirit, or if we do not explore or nourish our spirituality, we may find that life becomes a purely materialistic existence, lacking meaning and direction.

## SPLEEN

*Sophie Spleen*

The spleen is an organ located just under the rib cage on the left side of the body. It is part of the body's lymphatic system and it plays important role in the body's ability to manufacture antibodies that help resist infection. It also removes harmful microorganisms from the blood and gets rid of old blood cells. Before birth, the spleen manufactures red blood cells until after birth when the bone marrow can take over this process.

At the psycho-emotional level, the spleen is to do with fending off antagonism or aggression from others. If we have difficulty rejecting the antagonistic behaviour of others, we can end up having problems with the spleen.

## STOMACH

*Sam and Sylvie Stomach, Burnie, George Gastric*

The stomach is an enlarged, J-shaped, sac-like canal beneath the ribs and its main job is to digest proteins. It produces gastric enzymes, the most important of which is pepsin, which breaks down protein into smaller peptide fragments. The stomach also produces hydrochloric acid to help break down food into a liquid called chyme. Food is digested in the stomach for several hours, after which the chyme is slowly transported from the pylorus (end portion of the stomach) through a sphincter or valve and into the small intestine, where further digestion and nutrient absorption occurs.

At the psycho-emotional level, the stomach is to do with our mental state and with breaking down the details and scenarios of life so that we can work with them. If we have digestive or stomach problems, it normally means that we're having trouble processing life—figuring out what's going on, how we feel about any given situation and how we want to deal with it.

## TASTE BUDS

*Taste Buddies*

Taste buds are small structures on the upper surface of the tongue, soft palate, upper esophagus and epiglottis that provide information about the taste of food being eaten. The human tongue has about 10,000 taste buds and they detect the five elements of taste perception: salty, sour, bitter, sweet and savoury.

## THYMUS

The thymus is a duct-less gland in the upper part of the chest cavity. It is most active during puberty, after which it shrinks in size and activity and is replaced with fat. The thymus plays an important role in the development of the immune system in early life, and its cells form a part of the body's normal immune system. At the psycho-emotional level, the thymus is to do with taking aggressive action to protect ourselves from external invading forces, so that we are not diminished or overpowered by others.

## THYROID

The thyroid is a small, butterfly-shaped gland at the back of the neck beneath the Adam's apple. It produces thyroid hormones that control metabolism and influence every organ, tissue and cell in the body. These hormones also control heart rate, body weight, body temperature, energy level, muscle strength and menstrual regularity. There are two main types of thyroid malfunction: hypothyroidism (i.e., the thyroid does not produce enough thyroid hormone), which produces nervousness, decreased menstrual flow, weight loss and irregular heartbeat, and hyperthyroidism (i.e., the thyroid produces too much thyroid hormone), which increases all the reactions that occur in the body and results in fatigue, sluggishness, weakness, intolerance to cold, weight gain, depression, irritability, dry skin, coarse/dry hair, hair loss, muscle cramps and confusion/forgetfulness.

At the psycho-emotional level, the thyroid is to do with correcting injustices and speaking out when something doesn't feel morally or ethically right.

## TONGUE

The strongest muscle in the body, the tongue is a fleshy, movable organ, attached to the floor of the mouth. It is the principal organ of taste, an aid in chewing and swallowing, and an important organ of speech.

At the psycho-emotional level, the tongue represents our ability to mull things over and decide what tastes right. It relates to choice, since much of what we eat is determined by our taste buds and the flavours that we enjoy. Like our sense of smell, our sense of taste can often tell us which foods to avoid and which to favour.

## TOXINS

A toxin is any substance that is damaging to the health of the body. Toxins can come in the form of food additives, chemicals, pesticides, preservatives, artificial flavouring (such as MSG), colouring or sweeteners, vaccinations, drugs, medication, exhaust fumes, cigarette smoke, aerosol sprays, cosmetics, dental amalgams or anything else that the body cannot process effectively without harmful side-effects or byproducts.

## VILLI

Villi are tiny, finger-like projections that line the wall of the small intestine and are responsible for the absorption of nutrients. Circulating blood then carries these nutrients around the body.

## VITAMINS

Vitamins are a group of substances that occur naturally in certain foods and are essential to life. They contribute to good health by regulating the metabolism and assisting the biochemical processes that release energy from digested food. Most vitamins cannot be made by the body, but are found naturally in foods obtained from plants and animals. Vitamins are either water-soluble (such as vitamin C and the B complex, which is made up of B1 (thiamin), B2 (riboflavin), niacin, B6 (pyridoxine), folic acid, B12 (methylcobalamine), biotin and pantothenic acid) or fat-soluble (vitamins A, D, E and K). Most water-soluble vitamins travel through the bloodstream, acting as catalysts and coenzymes in metabolic processes and energy transfer. Whatever is not needed is excreted fairly rapidly in the urine. Fat-soluble vitamins are necessary for the function or structural integrity of specific body tissues and membranes and are stored in the fat tissues and in the liver until needed. An inadequate diet or problems with vitamin absorption can result in vitamin deficiencies, which can, in turn, lead to particular conditions or diseases. A vitamin D deficiency, for example, can result in osteoporosis or rickets, whereas a vitamin A deficiency can cause night blindness.

# Also available from Olga
### www.olgasheean.com

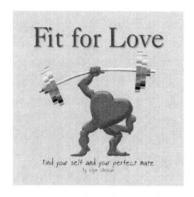

## Fit for Love—find your self and your perfect mate

This is a practical, power-packed illustrated workbook that takes readers on a journey of self-discovery, healing and empowerment. Filled with exercises, illustrations, tips and practical guidance, this book enables you to identify and transform the negative programming that's preventing you from having the love and fulfillment you seek.

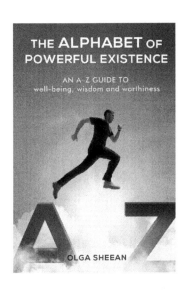

## The Alphabet of Powerful Existence—an A-Z guide to well-being, wisdom and worthiness

This is a practical guide to self-empowerment, featuring 52 themes (one for every week of the year) and offering simple, transformative steps for resolving conflict, positively reprogramming your mind, making powerful choices, and creating more love, money, ease, success and fulfillment in your life. Upgrade your relationships, finances and business; fill in your 'missing pieces'; activate your creativity; and enhance your self-worth and personal magnetism.

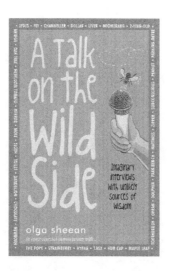

## A Talk on the Wild Side: imaginary interviews with unlikely sources of wisdom

Ever shared laughs with a hyena, chatted up a strawberry, or had a chinwag with a boomerang? Forget about all those gurus out there, telling you how to live your life. Wisdom is all around you, available in the most unlikely places—from dinosaurs to dandelions, mattresses to parking metres, popes to peanuts, toothbrushes to toilets, and plenty of other wiseguys you've never talked to before. *A Talk on the Wild Side* is a collection of outrageous conversations, filled with irreverent insights, off-the-wall humour, and a surprising number of salient truths. Life will never be the same again—and you'll find yourself talking to the strangest things. (Just don't let anyone see you doing it.)

# Consultations, coaching and training

## The ultimate operating system for humans

Learn a unique system for decoding your circumstances and mastering your business, relationships, finances, health and career. Practical, powerful and fast-acting, this system is the key to personal and professional fulfillment. E-mail Olga to arrange a complimentary Skype/phone chat, and find out how to powerfully manifest more love, money, ease, success and fulfillment in your life. The following coaching/counselling options are available, among others:

### Empowerment Intensive

A mini-workshop in itself, addressing emotional and relationship issues as well as any environmental or work-related factors that may be affecting your health, happiness or success. Includes a copy of *Fit for Love*, a recording of the session, a written summary and specific homework for creating practical, positive change.

### The Commitment Combo

Break free of old patterns and permanently resolve your emotional and personal issues, with ongoing support, at a very favourable rate. Includes a two-hour intensive and three one-hour sessions scheduled in accordance with your needs and progress.

### The Life-Changer—a power-packed three-month programme

A truly life-changing course providing personalized, intensive coaching and ongoing support designed to create deep and lasting breakthroughs in your life.

**Visit http://www.olgasheean.com for more info.**

# About Olga

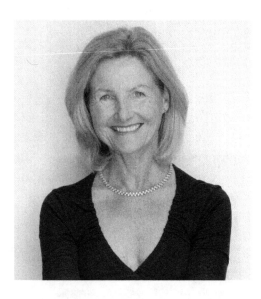

Olga Sheean is an author, empowerment coach, relationship therapist, and creative catalyst for lovership and leadership. She has developed a powerful system for resolving life's challenges, based on an understanding of the power and impact of our subconscious programming.

Her unique system shows individuals how to identify and transform their subconscious programming, which, in turn, transforms their circumstances—resulting in healthy, enlightened relationships, financial prosperity, and greater fulfillment. Tapping into universal principles, it is the ultimate approach to decoding life's scenarios and making sense of our world.

Olga's personalized programmes encompass health, lifestyle, career, personal growth, finances, relationships and whatever else may be a factor in an individual's success or fulfillment.

Olga developed her proprietary processes over 20 years of training, research and private practice in interpersonal dynamics, the body-mind connection, intuitive healing, conflict resolution and the powerful impact of negative subconscious programming. She works internationally, offering private consultations, Life-Changer intensives, Star-Smart programmes for actors and celebrities, Dream Teams, Empowerment Intensives and online training, dedicated to helping people enhance their relationships, health, career, finances and happiness quotient.

Her first book, *Fit for Love: find your self and your perfect mate*, is a power-packed illustrated workbook that takes readers on a journey of self-discovery, healing and empowerment. Olga is also the author of *The Alphabet of Powerful Existence* and *A Talk on the Wild Side—imaginary interviews with unlikely sources of wisdom*.

As a professional writer and editor with 25 years' experience, Olga has written over 250 articles and feature stories on human dynamics, relationships, empowerment, the environment, holistic lifestyles, healing, personal growth, nutrition and popular psychology, and has been a regular feature writer and columnist for magazines in Ireland, Canada, the States and Australia. A magazine editor for six years, she also established Berkana Books—a self-publishing company that produced non-fiction, self-help titles. Olga has also worked as a photo-journalist and editor for WWF International in Switzerland and as an editor for the United Nations in Geneva. She currently co-operates InsideOut Media—a self-publishing company for non-fiction titles that inspire, uplift and empower.

She is passionate about helping people grow, discover their true selves, and create love and magic in their lives.